High-Yield™ Biostatistics

UNIVERSITY BOOKSTORE
621 W LOMBARD STREET
BALTIMORE, MD 21201

10/11/00 3:53PM Op:001727 Trn. 0422438

ITEM NUMBER	PRICE	QTY	TOTAL
091	.95	1	
CONVENIENCE			.95
0683035660	15.95	1	
GLASER/HIGH YIELD			15.95

SUB-TOTAL   16.90
5 % SALES TAX   .85
TOTAL SALE   17.75

VISA/MASTERCARD   17.75

CHANGE   .00

ALL TEXTBOOKS ARE NON RETURNABLE
MERCHANDISE RETURNABLE WITHIN ONE WEEK
CONDITION AS PURCHASE AND WITH RECEIPT.

```
DATE 10100639303  TIME
10/11/00 0000000000  15:10

UNIV OF MARYLAND/BALT #639
        BALTIMORE, MD


TRAN #              AUTH
739                 11744
        SALE

ACCT. NUMBER        EXP
4305873960065534    0803


DESC_____


  TOTAL $          17.75

X_____
 SIGNATURE
      JOHN C GREENAWALT

THANK YOU FOR SHOPPING WITH US

   TOP COPY-MERCHANT
   BOTTOM COPY-CUSTOMER
```

10/11/00 3:23PM Op.001727 Trm. 0422438
VISA/MASTERCARD $17.75

High-Yield™ Biostatistics

Anthony N. Glaser, M.D., Ph.D., C. Psychol.
Medical University of South Carolina
Charleston, South Carolina

Williams & Wilkins
BALTIMORE • PHILADELPHIA • HONG KONG
LONDON • MUNICH • SYDNEY • TOKYO
A Waverly Company

Williams & Wilkins

Managing Editor: Amy G. Dinkel
Production Coordinator: Peter J. Carley
Compositor: Christopher O'Callaghan

Copyright © 1995
Williams & Wilkins
Suite 5025
Rose Tree Corporate Center–Bldg. II
1400 N. Providence Road
Media, PA 19063-2043 USA

Printed in the United States of America

ISBN 0-683-03566-5

97 98
2 3 4 5 6 7 8 9 10

To my wife, Marlene

Contents

Preface

Biostatistics is a course that most people dislike and try to scrape by on—often because it is taught by a statistician who assumes that everyone is adept at mathematics and can cope with blackboards full of formulae and equations. However, today's medical students will not, for the most part, become producers of research (and those who do will undoubtedly seek the advice of professional statisticians when designing their studies). On the other hand, all will become consumers of research and will need to understand the inferential statistical principles behind the reports that they read. Consequently, while this book does not pretend to be an in-depth statistics textbook (which few medical students have the need, the time, or the desire for), it aims to be more than a set of notes to be memorized for the purpose of examinations.

High-Yield Biostatistics explains concepts, provides examples, and also contains review exercises for the more difficult material in the first three chapters. Unlike other biostatistics books, it covers the complete range of biostatistics material that can be expected to appear on the USMLE Step 1, without going beyond that range.

The term "high yield" has become something of a buzzword among students. Its use here reflects that the core of information presented in *High-Yield Biostatistics* will be tested on the "Boards." The book contains little extraneous information, although the material does tread beyond the irreducible minimum in some instances.

For the more inquisitive reader, a small amount of additional material is presented in endnotes following each chapter, but this information is neither necessary for a general understanding of the material nor to answer USMLE questions.

If you have any suggestions for changes or improvements to this book, or if you find a biostatistics question on Step 1 that this book does not equip you to answer, please drop me a line.

Anthony N. Glaser

1

Descriptive Statistics

Statistical methods fall into two broad areas: **descriptive statistics** and **inferential statistics**.

Descriptive statistics merely describe, organize, or summarize data (such as the mean blood pressure of a group of patients, or the ratio of male to female alcoholics); they refer only to the actual data available.

Inferential statistics involve making inferences that go beyond the actual data. They typically involve inductive reasoning (i.e., generalizing to a population after having observed only a sample).

POPULATIONS, SAMPLES, AND ELEMENTS

A **population** is the universe about which an investigator wishes to draw conclusions; it need not consist of people. For the purposes of this book, patients in a hospital are discussed. A population refers to observations related to patients. If an investigator wants to know the plasma levels of a drug in a group of patients, the population consists of the patients' plasma levels, not the patients themselves.

A **sample** is a subset of the population—the part that is actually being observed or studied. Because researchers rarely can study whole populations, inferential statistics are almost always needed to draw conclusions about a population when only a sample has actually been studied.

A single observation is an **element**, denoted by X. The number of elements in a population is denoted by N, and the number of elements in a sample by n. A population therefore consists of all the elements from X_1 to X_N, and a sample consists of n of these N elements.

Most samples used in biomedical research are **probability samples**, samples in which the researcher can specify the probability of each population element being included. Probability samples permit the use of inferential statistics, whereas nonprobability samples allow only descriptive statistics to be used. There are four basic kinds of probability samples: **simple random samples**, **stratified random samples**, **cluster samples**, and **systematic samples**.

Simple random samples

The simple random sample is the simplest probability sample. It is a sample drawn so that every element in the population has an equal probability of being included. Note that a random sample is defined by the *method of drawing the sample*, not by the outcome.

1

A sample is **representative** if it closely resembles the population from which it is drawn. All types of random samples tend to be representative, but they cannot guarantee representativeness. Nonrepresentative samples can cause serious problems.

A classic example of a nonrepresentative sample is an opinion poll taken before the 1936 United States Presidential Election. On the basis of a very large sample (more than two million people), it was predicted that Alfred Landon would achieve a landslide victory over Franklin Delano Roosevelt—but the result was the opposite. The problem was that the sample was drawn from records of telephone and automobile ownership—and people who owned such items in this Depression year were not at all representative of the electorate as a whole.

A sample or a result demonstrates relative **bias** if it consistently errs in a particular direction. For example, in drawing a sample of 10 from a population consisting of 500 white people and 500 black people, a sampling method that consistently produces samples in which there are more than five white people would be biased. Biased samples are therefore unrepresentative; true randomization is proof against bias.

Stratified random samples

In a stratified random sample, the population is first divided into relatively internally homogeneous strata, or groups, from which random samples are then drawn. This stratification results in greater representativeness. For example, instead of drawing one sample of 10 people from a total population consisting of 500 black and 500 white people, two random samples of five could be taken from each racial group (or stratum) separately, thus guaranteeing the racial representativeness of the resulting overall sample of 10.

Cluster samples

Cluster samples may be used when it is too expensive or laborious to draw a simple random or stratified random sample. For example, in a survey of medical students in the United States, an investigator might start by selecting a random set of groups or "clusters"—such as a random set of 10 medical schools in the United States. In cluster sampling the clusters are sampled randomly, and all members of the cluster are sampled. This method is much more economical and practical than trying to take a random sample directly from the widely scattered population of all medical students in the United States.

Systematic samples

A systematic sample involves choosing elements in a systematic way—such as selecting every fifth patient admitted to a hospital, or every third infant born in a given area. This type of sampling provides the equivalent of a simple random sample without actually using randomization.

PROBABILITY

The **probability** of an event is a quantitative measure of the proportion of all possible, equally likely outcomes that are favorable to the event; it is denoted by p. Probabilities are usually expressed as decimal fractions, not as percentages, and must lie between zero (zero probability) and one (absolute certainty). The probability of an event cannot be negative. Probability of an event can be expressed as a ratio of the number of likely outcomes to the number of possible outcomes.

For example, if a fair coin were tossed an infinite number of times, heads would appear on 50% of the trials; therefore, the probability of heads, or *p* (heads), is .50. If a random sample of 10 people were drawn an infinite number of times from a population of 100 people, each person would be included in the sample 10% of the time; therefore, *p* (being included in any one sample) is .10.

The probability of an event *not* occurring is equal to one minus the probability that it will occur; this is denoted by **q**. In the above example, the probability of any one person *not* being included in any one sample, (*q*), is therefore (1 − *p*) = (1 − .10) = .90.

> The USMLE will require familiarity with the three main methods of calculating probabilities: the addition rule, the multiplication rule, and the binomial distribution.

Addition rule

The **addition rule** of probability states that the probability of any *one* of several particular events occurring is equal to the sum of their individual probabilities, *provided* the events are mutually exclusive (i.e., they cannot *both* happen).

Because the probability of picking a diamond card from a deck of cards is 0.25, and the probability of picking a heart card is also 0.25, this rule states that the probability of picking one card that is either a diamond or a heart is 0.25 + 0.25 = 0.50. Because no card can be both a diamond and a heart, these events meet the requirement of mutual exclusiveness.

Multiplication rule

The **multiplication rule** of probability states that the probability of two or more statistically independent events *all* occurring is equal to the product of their individual probabilities.

If the lifetime probability of a person developing cancer is 0.25, and the lifetime probability of developing schizophrenia is 0.01, the lifetime probability that a person might have *both* cancer *and* schizophrenia is 0.25 × 0.01 = .0025, *provided* that the two illnesses are independent—in other words, that having one illness neither increases nor decreases the risk of having the other.

Binomial distribution

The probability that a *specific combination of mutually exclusive independent events* will occur can be determined by the use of the **binomial distribution**. A binomial distribution is one in which there are only two possibilities, such as yes/no, male/female, healthy/sickly. If an experiment has exactly two possible outcomes (one of which is generally termed "success"), and the probability of success is *p*, the binomial distribution gives the probability of obtaining exactly *r* successes in *n* independent trials. The formula for the binomial distribution does not need to be learned or used for the purposes of the USMLE, but its use must be understood.

A typical medical use of the binomial distribution is in genetic counseling. Inheritance of a disorder such as Tay-Sachs disease follows a binomial distribution: there are two possible events (inheriting the disease or not inheriting it) that are mutually exclusive (one person cannot both have and not have the disease), and the possibilities are independent (if one child in a family inherits the disorder, this does not affect the chance of another child inheriting it).

A physician could therefore use the binomial distribution to inform a couple who are carriers of the disease how probable it is that some specific combination of events might occur—such as the probability that if they are to have two children, *neither* will inherit the disease. Probability in a binomial distribution is calculated by the following formula:

$$p = \frac{n!}{r!(n-r)!} \; p^r (1-p)^{n-r}$$

where: n is the number of trials (in this case, the number of children);

p is the probability of the specified event occurring (in this case, the probability that any one child will inherit the disease, which is .25);

r is the number of times the specified event occurs (in this case, zero, as it is specified that no child shall have the disease), $r = 0$; and

$n!$ is "n factorial" or "n prime," the product of n times every number from n to 1 (e.g., if $n = 5$, $n! = 5 \times 4 \times 3 \times 2 \times 1$). By convention, $0! = 1$.

In this example, therefore, the probability is

$$p = \frac{2!}{0!(2-0)!} 0.25^0 (1-0.25)^{2-0}$$

$$= \frac{2!}{2!} \times 0.75^2$$

$$= 0.5625$$

The probability that both of this couple's planned two children will be free of the disease is therefore .5625.

Note: Try examples where $r \neq 0$ to understand the application of the binomial distribution.

TYPES OF DATA

The choice of an appropriate statistical technique depends on the type of data in question. Data will always form one of the four **scales of measurement**: nominal, ordinal, interval, or ratio. Use the mnemonic NOIR to remember these scales in order. Data may also be characterized as being discrete or continuous.

Nominal

Nominal scale data are divided into qualitative categories or groups, such as male/female, black/white, urban/suburban/rural. There is no implication of order or ratio. Nominal data that fall into only two groups are called dichotomous data.

Ordinal

Ordinal scale data can be placed in a meaningful order (e.g., students may be ranked 1st/2nd/3rd in their class). However, there is no information about the size of the interval—no conclusion can be drawn about whether the difference between the first and second students is the same as the difference between the second and third.

Interval

Interval scale data have the same quality as do ordinal data, in that they can be placed in a meaningful order. In addition these data have meaningful intervals between items, which are usually measured quantities. For example, on the Celsius scale the difference between 100° and 90° is the same as the difference between 50° and 40°. However, because interval scales do not have an absolute zero, ratios of scores are not meaningful: 100°C is *not* twice as hot as 50°C, because 0°C does not indicate a complete absence of heat.

Ratio

A ratio scale has the same properties as an interval scale; but because it has an absolute zero, meaningful ratios do exist. Most biomedical variables form a ratio scale: weight in grams or pounds, time in seconds or days, blood pressure in millimeters of mercury, and pulse rate are all ratio scale data. The only ratio scale of temperature is the Kelvin scale, in which zero degrees indicates an absolute absence of heat, just as a zero pulse rate indicates an absolute lack of heartbeat. Therefore, it is correct to say that a pulse rate of 120 is twice as fast as a pulse rate of 60.

Discrete

Discrete variables can take only certain values, and none in between. For example, the number of patients in a hospital may be 178 or 179, but it cannot be any value between these two. The number of syringes used in a clinic on any given day may increase or decrease only by units of one.

Continuous

Continuous variables may take any value (typically between certain limits). Most biomedical variables are continuous (e.g., a patient's weight, height, age, and blood pressure). However, the process of measuring or reporting continuous variables will reduce them to a discrete variable; blood pressure may be reported to the nearest whole millimeter of mercury, weight to the nearest pound, and so on.

FREQUENCY DISTRIBUTIONS

A set of unorganized data is difficult to digest and understand. Consider a study of the serum cholesterol levels of a sample of 200 men: a list of the 200 levels would be of little value in itself. A simple first step toward organizing the data is to list all the possible values between the highest and the lowest in order, recording the frequency (f) with which each score occurs. This forms a **frequency distribution**. If the highest serum cholesterol level were 260 mg/dl, and the lowest were 161 mg/dl, the frequency distribution might be as shown in Table 1-1.

Table 1-1

Score	f	Score	f	Score	f	Score	f	Score	f
260	1	240	2	220	4	200	3	180	0
259	0	239	1	219	2	199	0	179	2
258	1	238	2	218	1	198	1	178	1
257	0	237	0	217	3	197	3	177	0
256	0	236	3	216	4	196	2	176	0
255	0	235	1	215	5	195	0	175	0
254	1	234	2	214	3	194	3	174	1
253	0	233	2	213	4	193	1	173	0
252	1	232	4	212	6	192	0	172	0
251	1	231	2	211	5	191	2	171	1
250	0	230	3	210	8	190	2	170	1
249	2	229	1	209	9	189	1	169	1
248	1	228	0	208	1	188	2	168	0
247	1	227	2	207	9	187	1	167	0
246	0	226	3	206	8	186	0	166	0
245	1	225	3	205	6	185	2	165	1
244	2	224	2	204	8	184	1	164	0
243	3	223	1	203	4	183	1	163	0
242	2	222	2	202	5	182	1	162	0
241	1	221	1	201	4	181	1	161	1

Grouped frequency distributions

Table 1-1 is an unwieldy presentation of data. These data can be made more manageable by creating a **grouped frequency distribution**, as shown in Table 1-2. Individual scores are grouped (between seven and twenty groups are usually appropriate). Each group of scores encompasses an equal **class interval**. In this example there are 10 groups with a class interval of 10 (161 to 170, 171 to 180, and so on).

Table 1-2

Interval	Frequency f	Relative f % rel f	Cumulative f % cum f
251–260	5	2.5	100.0
241–250	13	6.5	97.5
231–240	19	9.5	91.0
221–230	18	9.0	81.5
211–220	38	19.0	72.5
201–210	72	36.0	53.5
191–200	14	7.0	17.5
181–190	12	6.0	10.5
171–180	5	2.5	4.5
161–170	4	2.0	2.0

Relative frequency distributions

As Table 1-2 shows, a grouped frequency distribution can be transformed into a **relative frequency distribution**, which shows the *percentage* of elements that fall within each class interval. The relative frequency of elements in any given class interval is found by dividing f, the frequency (or number of elements) in that class interval, by n (the sample size, which in this case is 200); by multiplying the result by 100, the results are converted into a percentage. Therefore, this distribution shows, for example, that 19% of this sample had serum cholesterol levels between 211 and 220 mg/dl.

Cumulative frequency distributions

Table1-2 also shows a **cumulative frequency distribution**. This is also expressed as a percentage; it shows the percentage of elements lying *within and below* each class interval. Note that although a group may be called the 211–220 group, for example, this group actually encompasses the range of scores that lie from 210.5 up to and including 220.5. The figure of 220.5 is therefore called the **exact upper limit** of the group.

The relative frequency column shows that 2% of the distribution lies in the 161–170 group and 2.5% lies in the 171–180 group; therefore, a total of 4.5% of the distribution lies at or below a score of 180.5, as shown by the cumulative frequency column in Table 1-2. A further 6% of the distribution lies in the 181–190 group; therefore, a total of (2 + 2.5 + 6) = 10.5% lies at or below a score of 190.5. A man with a serum cholesterol level of 190 mg/dl can be told that roughly 10% of this sample had lower levels than his, whereas approximately 90% had scores above his. Note that the cumulative frequency of the highest group (251–260) must be 100, showing that 100% of the distribution lies at or below a score of 260.5.

Graphical presentations of frequency distributions

Frequency distributions are often presented in graphical forms, most commonly as **histograms**. Figure 1-1 is a histogram of the grouped frequency distribution shown in Table 1-2; the **abscissa** (X or horizontal axis) shows the grouped scores, whereas the **ordinate** (Y or vertical axis) shows the frequencies.

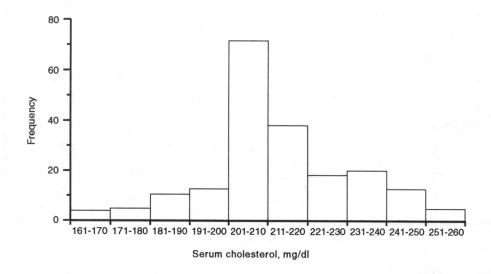

Figure 1-1

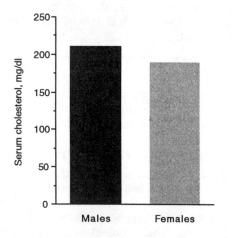

Figure 1-2

To display nominal scale data, a **bar graph** is typically used. For example, if a group of 100 men had a mean serum cholesterol value of 212, and a group of 100 women had a mean level of 185, the means of these two groups could be presented as a bar graph, as shown in Figure 1-2.

Bar graphs are identical to frequency histograms, except that each rectangle on the graph is clearly separated from the others by a space, demonstrating that the data form separate categories (such as male and female) rather than continuous groups.

For ratio or interval scale data, a frequency distribution may be drawn as a **frequency polygon**, in which the midpoints of each class interval are joined by straight lines, as shown in Figure 1-3.

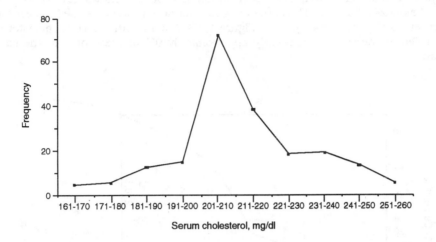

Figure 1-3

A cumulative frequency distribution can also be presented graphically as a polygon, as shown in Figure 1-4A. Cumulative frequency polygons typically form a characteristic S-shaped curve known as an **ogive**, which the curve in Figure 1-4A approximately resembles.

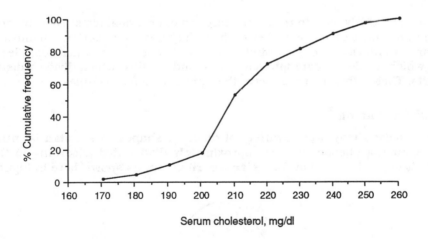

Figure 1-4A

Centiles and other quantiles

The cumulative frequency polygon and the cumulative frequency distribution both demon-strate the concept of **centile** (or **percentile**) **rank**. This is a descriptive statistic that states the percentage of observations that fall below any particular score. In the case of a grouped frequency distribution, such as the one in Table 1-2, centile ranks state the percentage of observations that fall within or below any given class interval. Centile ranks provide a way of giving information about one individual score in relation to all the other scores in a distribution.

For example, the cumulative frequency distribution in Table 1-2 shows that 91% of the observations fall below 240.5 mg/dl. The figure of 240.5 therefore represents the 91st centile (which can be written as C_{91}), as shown here in Figure 1-4B. A man with a serum cholesterol level of 240 mg/dl lies at the 91st centile—only approximately 9% of the scores in the sample are higher than his.

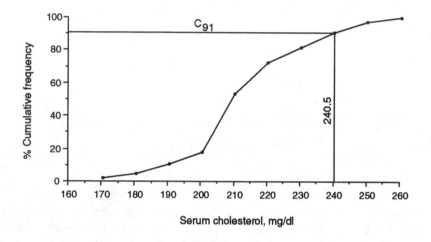

Figure 1-4B

Centile ranks are widely used in reporting scores on educational tests. They are one member of a family of values called **quantiles**, each of which divides a distribution into a number of equal parts. Centiles divide a distribution into 100 equal parts; other quantiles include **quartiles**, which divide the data into four parts, and **deciles**, which divide a distribution into 10 parts. These other quantiles serve the same function as centiles.

The normal distribution

Frequency polygons may take a variety of different shapes. A substantial number of naturally occurring phenomena are approximately distributed according to the symmetrical, bell-shaped normal or **Gaussian distribution**, as shown here in Figure 1-5.

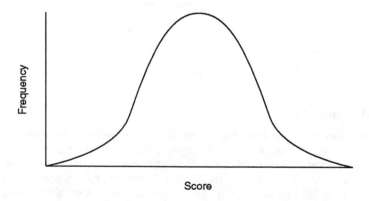

Figure 1-5

Skewed, J-shaped, and bimodal distributions

Other frequency distributions are shown in Figure 1-6. Asymmetrical frequency distributions are **skewed** distributions. **Positively** (or **right**) **skewed** distributions and **negatively** (or **left**) **skewed** distributions can be identified by the location of the *tail* of the curve (not by the location of the hump—a common error). Positively skewed distributions have a relatively large number of low scores and a small number of very high scores, whereas negatively skewed distributions have a large number of high scores and a relatively small number of low scores.

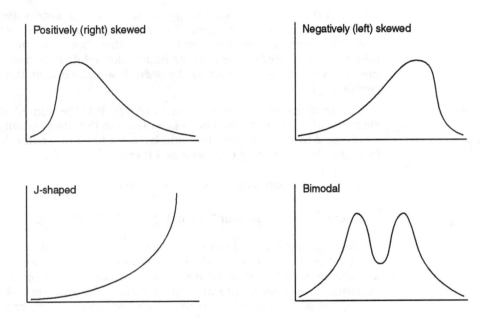

Figure 1-6

Figure 1-6 also shows a **J-shaped** distribution and a **bimodal** distribution. Bimodal distributions may be a combination of two underlying normal distributions, such as the heights of a large number of men and women—each sex forms its own normal distribution around a different central mode.

MEASURES OF CENTRAL TENDENCY

Researchers usually characterize an entire distribution by one typical figure that represents all the observations. Such figures are **measures of central tendency**; these measures include the **mode**, the **median**, and the **mean**:

Mode   The mode is the observed value that occurs with the greatest frequency. It is determined by simple inspection of the frequency distribution. If two scores both occur with the greatest frequency, the distribution is **bimodal**; if more than two scores occur with the greatest frequency, the distribution is **multimodal**. The mode is sometimes symbolized by *Mo*. *The mode is totally uninfluenced by small numbers of extreme scores in a distribution.*

Median

The median is the figure that divides the frequency distribution in half when all the scores are listed in order. When a distribution has an odd number of elements, the median is therefore the middle one; when it has an even number of elements, the median lies halfway between the two middle scores (i.e., it is the average or mean of the two middle scores).

For example, in a distribution consisting of the elements 6, 9, 15, 17, 24, the median would be 15; but if the distribution were 6, 9, 15, 17, 24, 29, the median would be 16 (the average of 15 and 17).

Note that the median responds only to the number of scores above it and below it, not to their value. The median is *insensitive to small numbers of extreme scores in a distribution*; therefore, it is a very useful measure of central tendency for highly skewed distributions. The median is sometimes symbolized by **Mdn**. It is the same as the 50th centile (C_{50}).

Mean

The mean is commonly known as the average. It is the sum of all the elements divided by the number of elements in the distribution. It is symbolized by μ in a population, and by $\overline{X}$ ("x-bar") in a sample. The formulas for calculating the mean are therefore

$$\mu = \frac{\sum X}{N} \text{ in a population, and } \overline{X} = \frac{\sum X}{n} \text{ in a sample}$$

where $\sum$ is "the sum of," so that $\sum X = X_1 + X_2 + X_3 + ... X_n$

Unlike other measures of central tendency, the mean responds to the exact value of every score in the distribution, and unlike the median and the mode, it is very sensitive to extreme scores. As a result, it is not usually an appropriate measure for characterizing very skewed distributions. On the other hand, it has the desirable property that repeated samples drawn from the same population will tend to have very similar means; the mean is therefore the measure of central tendency that best resists the influence of fluctuation between different samples.

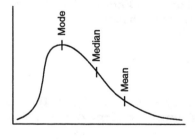

Figure 1-7

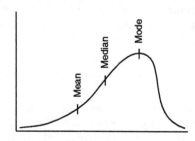

Figure 1-8

The relationship among the three measures of central tendency depends on the shape of the distribution. All three measures are identical in a unimodal symmetrical distribution (such as the normal distribution), but, in general, they differ in a skewed distribution. Figures 1-7 and 1-8 show positively and negatively skewed distributions, respectively. In both of these the mode is simply the most frequently occurring score; the mean is influenced by the relatively small number of very high or very low scores; and the median lies between the two, dividing the distribution into two equal halves (i.e., into two equal areas under the curve).

MEASURES OF VARIABILITY

Figure 1-9 shows two normal distributions, A and B; their means, modes, and medians are all identical, and, like all normal distributions, they are symmetrical and unimodal. But despite their similarities, these two distributions are obviously different—so to describe a normal distribution in terms of the three measures of central tendency alone is clearly inadequate.

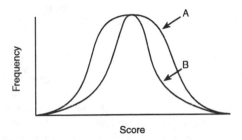

Figure 1-9

Although these two distributions have identical measures of central tendency, they differ in terms of their **variability**—the extent to which the scores are clustered together or scattered about. The scores forming distribution A are clearly more scattered than are those forming distribution B. Variability is a very important quality: if these two distributions represented the blood pressures of patients taking two different antihypertensive drugs, for example, then drug B would be the better medication, as fewer patients on this distribution have very high or very low blood pressures—even though the *mean* effect of drug B is the same as that of drug A.

There are three important measures of variability: **range**, **variance**, and **standard deviation**.

Range

The range is the simplest measure of variability. It is the difference between the lowest and the highest scores in the distribution. It therefore responds to these two scores only.

For example, in the distribution 6, 9, 15, 17, 24, the range is $(24 - 6) = 18$; but in the distribution 6, 9, 15, 17, 24, 318, the range is $(318 - 6) = 312$.

Variance (and deviation scores)

Calculating variance (and standard deviation) involves the use of **deviation scores**. The deviation score of a given element is found by subtracting the mean of the distribution from the element. A deviation score is symbolized by the letter x (as opposed to X, which symbolizes an element).

For example, in a distribution with a mean of 16, an element of 23 would have a deviation score of $(23 - 16) = 7$. On the same distribution, an element of 11 would have a deviation score of $(11 - 16) = -5$.

When calculating deviation scores for all the elements in a distribution, the results can be verified by checking that the sum of the deviation scores for all the elements in the distribution is zero; i.e., $\Sigma x = 0$.

The **variance** of a distribution is the mean of the squares of all the deviation scores in the distribution. The variance is therefore obtained by finding the deviation score for each element, squaring each of these deviation scores (thus eliminating minus signs), and then obtaining their mean in the usual way—by adding them all up and then dividing them by their number.

Variance is symbolized by σ^2 for a population and by S^2 for a sample. Thus,

$$\sigma^2 = \frac{\sum(X-\mu)^2}{N} \text{ or } \frac{\sum x^2}{N} \text{ in a population, and } S^2 = \frac{\sum(X-\overline{X})^2}{n} \text{ or } \frac{\sum x^2}{n} \text{ in a sample.}[1]$$

Variance is sometimes known as **mean square**. Note that variance is expressed in squared units of measurement, limiting its usefulness as a descriptive term.

Standard deviation

The standard deviation remedies this problem: it is the *square root* of the variance, so it is expressed in the same units of measurement as the original data. The symbols for standard deviation are therefore the same as the symbols for variance, but without being raised to the power of two. Therefore, the standard deviation of a population is σ, and the standard deviation of a sample is S. Standard deviation is sometimes written as *SD*.

Although standard deviation is not intuitively meaningful at first sight, one useful rule of thumb states that when a distribution's standard deviation is greater than its mean, the mean is inadequate as a representative measure of central tendency.

The standard deviation is particularly useful in normal distributions, because *the proportion of elements in the normal distribution* (i.e., the proportion of the area under the curve) *is a constant for a given number of standard deviations above or below the mean of the distribution,* as shown in Figure 1-10.

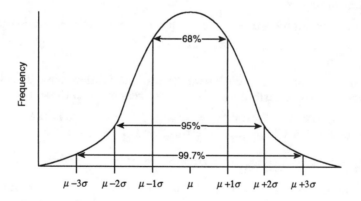

Figure 1-10

In Figure 1-10, approximately **68%** of the distribution falls within ± **1** standard deviation of the mean; **95%** of the distribution falls within ± **2** standard deviations of the mean; and **99.7%** of the distribution falls within ± **3** standard deviations of the mean.

---

*Because these proportions hold true for **every** normal distribution, they can be memorized.*

Therefore, if a population's resting heart rate is normally distributed with a mean of 70 and a standard deviation of 10, we can state what proportion of the population has a resting heart rate between certain limits.

As Figure 1-11 shows, because 68% of the distribution lies within approximately ±1 standard deviation of the mean, 68% of the population will have a resting heart rate between 60 and 80.

Similarly, 95% of the population will have a resting heart rate between approximately 70 ± (2 × 10) = 50 and 90 (i.e., within two standard deviations of the mean).

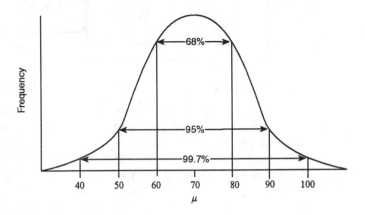

Figure 1-11

Z SCORES

The location of any element in a normal distribution can be expressed in terms of how many standard deviations it lies above or below the mean of the distribution. This is the **z score** of the element. If the element lies above the mean, it will have a positive z score, whereas if it lies below the mean, it will have a negative z score. A heart rate of 85 in the distribution shown in Figure 1-11 lies 1.5 standard deviations above the mean; it has a z score of +1.5. A heart rate of 65 lies 0.5 standard deviations below the mean; its z score is -0.5. The formula for calculating z scores is therefore

$$z = \frac{X - \mu}{\sigma}$$

Tables for z values

Tables of z values state what proportion of any normal distribution lies above *any* given z value, not just z values of ±1, 2, or 3. Table 1-3 is an abbreviated table of z values; it shows, for example, that .3085 (approximately 31%) of any normal distribution lies above a z value of +0.5. Because normal distributions are symmetrical, this also means that .3085 of the distribution lies *below* a z value of *minus* 0.5 (which corresponds to a heart rate of 65 in the population depicted in Figure 1-11); therefore, approximately 31% of this population has a heart rate of below 65. By subtracting this proportion from 1, it can be found that .6915, or approximately 69%, of the population has a heart rate of *above* 65.

Z values are standardized or normalized (for a distribution with mean = 1 and standard deviation = 0), as they allow scores on different normal distributions to be compared. For example, a person's heart rate and serum cholesterol level could be compared by means of their respective z values, provided that both these variables are elements in normal distributions.

Table 1-3

z	Area beyond z	z	Area beyond z
0.00	.5000	1.65	.0495
0.05	.4801	1.70	.0446
0.10	.4602	1.75	.0401
0.15	.4404	1.80	.0359
0.20	.4207	1.85	.0322
0.25	.4013	1.90	.0287
0.30	.3821	1.95	.0256
0.35	.3632	2.00	.0228
0.40	.3446	2.05	.0202
0.45	.3264	2.10	.0179
0.50	.3085	2.15	.0158
0.55	.2912	2.20	.0139
0.60	.2743	2.25	.0112
0.65	.2578	2.30	.0107
0.70	.2420	2.35	.0094
0.75	.2266	2.40	.0082
0.80	.2119	2.45	.0071
0.85	.1977	2.50	.0062
0.90	.1841	2.55	.0054
0.95	.1711	2.60	.0047
1.00	.1587	2.65	.0040
1.05	.1469	2.70	.0035
1.10	.1357	2.75	.0030
1.15	.1251	2.80	.0026
1.20	.1151	2.85	.0022
1.25	.1056	2.90	.0019
1.30	.0968	2.95	.0016
1.35	.0885	3.00	.0013
1.40	.0808	3.05	.0011
1.45	.0735	3.10	.0010
1.50	.0668	3.15	.0008
1.55	.0606	3.20	.0007
1.60	.0548	3.30	.0005

This table is not a complete listing of z scores. Full z score tables can be found in most statistics textbooks.

Instead of using z scores to find the proportion of a distribution corresponding to a particular score, the converse can also be done: using z scores to find the score that divides the distribution into specified proportions.

For example, if we want to know what heart rate divides the fastest-beating 5% of the population (i.e., the group at or above the 95th percentile) from the remaining 95%, we can use the z score table.

The table shows that the z score corresponding to this approximate division (the nearest figure shown in the tables is .0495, rather than exactly .05) is 1.65.

As shown in Figure 1-12, the corresponding heart rate therefore lies 1.65 standard deviations above the mean, i.e., it is equal to $\mu + 1.65\sigma =$ 70 + (1.65 × 10) = 86.5. So we can conclude that the fastest-beating 5% of this population has a heart rate above 86.5.

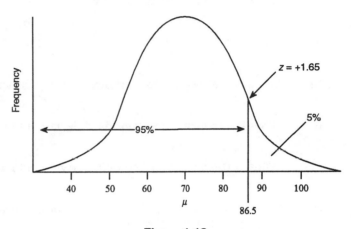

Figure 1-12

Note that the z score that divides the top 5% of the population from the remaining 95% is *not* approximately 2; although 95% of the distribution falls between approximately ± 2 standard deviations of the mean, this is the *middle* 95%, which leaves the remaining 5% split into two equal parts at the two tails of the distribution (remember—normal distributions are symmetrical)—so only 2.5% of the distribution falls more than 2 standard deviations *above* the mean, and another 2.5% falls more than 2 standard deviations *below* the mean.

Using z scores to specify probability

Z scores also allow us to specify the probability of a randomly picked element being above or below a particular score.

For example, if we know that 5% of the population has a heart rate above 86.5, then the probability of one randomly selected person from this population having a heart rate above 86.5 will be 5%, or .05.

Similarly, we can find the probability that a randomly picked person will have a heart rate of less than 50. Because 50 lies 2 standard deviations (i.e., 2 × 10) below the mean (70), it corresponds to a z score of -2, and we know that approximately 95% of the distribution lies within the limits $z = \pm 2$. Therefore, 5% of the distribution lies outside these limits, equally in each of the two tails of the distribution. Therefore, 2.5% of the distribution lies below 50, and the probability of a randomly selected person having a heart rate of less than 50 is 2.5%, or .025.

NOTE

[1] Some statisticians prefer to use a denominator of $n-1$ rather than n in the formula for sample variance. Both formulas are correct; using $n-1$ is preferred when the variance of a small sample is being used to estimate the variance of the population.

EXERCISES

1. If $\overline{X}$ = 40 and X = 45, what is x?

2. If $\overline{X}$ = 60 and X = 40, what is x?

3. If μ = 37 and X = 29, what is x?

4. What is the formula for variance in a sample?

5. What is the formula for variance in a population?

6. What is the formula for standard deviation in a sample?

7. What is the formula for standard deviation in a population?

8. What proportion of any normal distribution lies within approximately ±1σ of μ?

9. What proportion of any normal distribution lies within approximately ±2σ of μ?

10. What proportion of any normal distribution lies within approximately ±3σ of μ?

11. In a normal distribution, if μ = 10, σ = 2, and X = 12, what is the z score of X?

12. In a normal distribution, if μ = 10, σ = 2, and X = 6, what is the z score of X?

13. In a normal distribution, if μ = 10 and σ = 2, what proportion of the distribution falls between 8 and 12?

14. In a normal distribution, if μ = 100 and σ = 20, what proportion of the distribution falls between 60 and 140?

15. In a normal distribution, if μ = 50 and σ = 10, how likely is it that a randomly selected element will have a score above 70?

2

Inferential Statistics

At the end of the previous chapter, it was shown how z scores can be used to find the probability that a randomly chosen element will have a score of above or below a certain value. This requires that the population is normally distributed, and that both the population mean (μ) and the population standard deviation (σ) are known.

Most research, however, involves the opposite kind of problem: instead of using information about a *population* to draw conclusions or make predictions about a *sample*, the researcher usually wants to use the information provided by a *sample* to draw conclusions about a *population*. For example, a researcher might want to forecast the results of an election on the basis of an opinion poll, or predict the effectiveness of a new drug on all patients with a certain disease after it has been tested on only a small sample of patients.

STATISTICS AND PARAMETERS

In such problems the population mean and standard deviation, μ and σ, which are called the population **parameters**, are unknown; all that is known is the sample mean ($\overline{X}$) and the sample standard deviation (S)—these are called the sample **statistics**. The task of using a sample to draw conclusions about a population involves **inference**: going beyond the actual information that is available. Inferential statistics therefore involves using a statistic to estimate a parameter.

However, it is unlikely that a sample will be perfectly representative of the population from which it is drawn; that is, a statistic (such as the sample mean) will not exactly reflect its corresponding parameter (the population mean). For example, in a study of intelligence, if a sample is drawn from a population with a mean IQ of 100, the sample mean cannot be expected to be exactly 100; there will be **sampling error** that will cause the sample statistic to differ from the population parameter.

The random sampling distribution of means

Sampling error can be demonstrated by drawing a large number of random samples (of equal size) from the same population. The means of all these samples are not the same. Because of sampling error, they spread out to form a distribution that is called the **random sampling distribution of means**.

CENTRAL LIMIT THEOREM

The **central limit theorem** states that *the random sampling distribution of means will always tend to be normal, irrespective of the shape of the population distribution from which* *the samples were drawn.* Figure 2-1 is a random sampling distribution of means; even if the underlying population were distributed in a skewed or other non-normal fashion, the means of all the random samples drawn from it will always tend to form a normal distribution. Furthermore, the theorem states that the random sampling distribution of means will become closer to normal as the size of the samples increases.

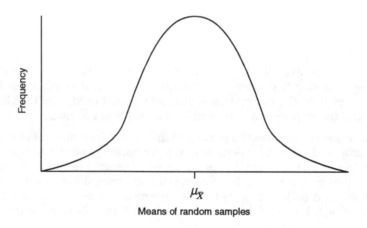

Figure 2-1

The theorem also states that the mean of the random sampling distribution of means (symbolized by $\mu_{\bar{x}}$, showing that it is the mean of the population of all the sample means) is equal to the mean of the original population; in other words, $\mu_{\bar{x}}$ is equal to μ.

In addition, the standard deviation of the random sampling distribution of means (symbolized by $\sigma_{\bar{x}}$, signifying that it is the standard deviation of the population of all the sample means) is equal to the population standard deviation (s) divided by the square root of the size of the samples. Therefore, the formula for the standard deviation of the random sampling distribution of means is

$$\sigma_{\bar{x}} = \frac{\sigma}{\sqrt{n}}$$

Standard error

The standard deviation of the random sampling distribution of means, $\sigma_{\bar{x}}$, has its own name: it is called the **standard error**, or the **standard error of the mean**, sometimes abbreviated as *SE* or *SEM*. *It is a measure of the extent to which the sample means deviate from the true population mean.* As its formula shows, it is dependent on the size of the samples: *standard error is inversely related to the square root of the sample size*, so that the larger n becomes, the more closely will the sample means represent the true population mean. This is the reason why the results of large studies or surveys are more trusted than the results of small ones.

Predicting the probability of drawing samples with a given mean

Because the random sampling distribution of means is by definition normal, investigators can use the known facts about normal distributions and z scores to predict the probability that a *sample* will have a *mean* of above or below a given value, provided, of course, that the sample is random. This is a step beyond what was possible in Chapter 1, where only the probability that *one element* would have a score of above or below a given value was predicted.

In addition, owing to the fact that the central limit theorem states that the random sampling distribution of means is normal even when the underlying population is not normally distributed, z scores can be used to make predictions irrespective of the shape of the underlying population distribution—provided, once again, that the sample is random.

Using the standard error

The method used to make a prediction about a sample mean is similar to the method used in Chapter 1 to make a prediction about a single element—it involves finding the z score corresponding to the value of interest. But instead of calculating the z score in terms of the number of *standard deviations* by which a given *single element* lies above or below the population mean, the z score is now calculated in terms of the number of *standard errors* by which a *sample mean* lies above or below the population mean; therefore, the previous formula

$$z = \frac{X - \mu}{\sigma} \quad \text{now becomes} \quad z = \frac{\overline{X} - \mu}{\sigma_{\overline{X}}}$$

For example, in a population with a mean resting heart rate of 70 and a standard deviation of 10, the probability that a random sample of 25 people will have a mean heart rate of above 75 can be found. The steps are:

1. Calculate the standard error: $\sigma_{\overline{X}} = \dfrac{\sigma}{\sqrt{n}} = \dfrac{10}{\sqrt{25}} = 2$

2. Calculate the z score of the sample mean: $z = \dfrac{\overline{X} - \mu}{\sigma_{\overline{X}}} = \dfrac{75 - 70}{2} = 2.5$

3. Find the proportion of the normal distribution that lies beyond this z score (2.5). Table 1-3 shows that the proportion of the normal distribution that lies above a z score of +2.5 is .0062. Therefore, the probability that a random sample of 25 people from this population will have a mean resting heart rate of above 75 is .0062.

Conversely, it is possible to find what random sample mean (n = 25) is so high that it would occur in only 5% or less of all samples (in other words, what random sample mean is so high that the probability of obtaining it is .05 or less):

Table 1-3 shows that the z score that divides the bottom .95 of the distribution from the top .05 is +1.65. This z score therefore corresponds to a heart rate of μ + 1.65 $\sigma_{\overline{X}}$ (the population mean plus 1.65 standard errors). Because the population mean is 70 and the standard error is 2, the heart rate is therefore 70 + (1.65 × 2), or 73.3. Figure 2-2 shows the relevant portions of the random sampling distribution of means; note that the appropriate z score is +1.65, not +2, because it refers to the *top .05* of the distribution, not the top .025 and the bottom .025 together.

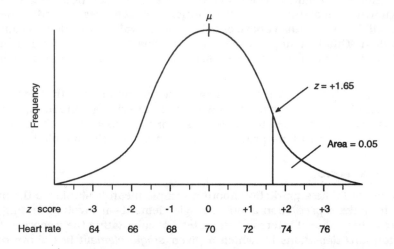

Figure 2-2

It is also possible to find the limits between which 95% of all possible random sample means would be expected to fall. As with any normal distribution, 95% of the random sampling distribution of means lies within approximately ±2 **standard errors of the population mean** (in other words, within $z = \pm 2$); therefore, 95% of all possible sample means must lie within approximately ±2 standard errors of the population mean.[1] Applying this to the distribution of resting heart rate, it is apparent that 95% of all possible random sample means will fall between the limits of $\mu \pm 2\ \sigma_{\bar{x}}$, that is, $70 \pm (2 \times 2)$, or 66 and 74.

ESTIMATING THE MEAN OF A POPULATION

So far it has been shown how z scores can be used to predict the probability that a random sample will have a mean of above or below a given value, irrespective of the shape of the underlying population distribution. It has been shown that 95% of all possible members of the population will lie within approximately ±2 (or, more exactly, ±1.96) standard errors of the population mean, and 95% of all such means will be within ± 2 standard errors of the mean.

Confidence limits

Logically, if the sample mean ($\bar{X}$) lies within ±1.96 standard errors of the population mean (μ) 95% (.95) of the time, then μ must lie within ±1.96 standard errors of $\bar{X}$ 95% of the time. These limits of ±1.96 standard errors are called the **confidence limits** (in this case, the 95% confidence limits). Finding the confidence limits involves the beginnings of inferential statistics because a sample statistic ($\bar{X}$) is used to estimate a population parameter (μ).

For example, if an investigator wants to find the true mean resting heart rate of a large population, it would be impractical to take the pulse of every person in the population. Instead, we can draw a random sample from the population and take the pulse of the people in the sample. Provided the sample is truly random, the investigator can be 95% confident that the true population mean lies within ±1.96 standard errors of the sample mean obtained.

Therefore, if the mean heart rate in the sample ($\overline{X}$) is 74 and $\sigma_{\overline{x}} = 2$, the investigator can be 95% certain that μ lies within 1.96 standard errors of 74, i.e., between 74 ± (1.96 × 2), or 70.08 and 77.92. This can be written as

$$C\,(70.08 \leq \mu \leq 77.92) = .95$$

This formula means that the confidence (C) with which the mean can be estimated to lie between 70.08 and 77.92 is .95. Note, however, that the best *single* estimate of the population mean is still the sample mean, 74—after all, it is the only piece of actual data on which an estimate can be based.

In general, confidence limits are equal to the sample mean plus or minus the z score obtained from the table (for the appropriate level of confidence) multiplied by the standard error:

$$\text{Confidence limits} = \overline{X} \pm z\,\sigma_{\overline{x}}$$

Therefore, 95% confidence limits, which are the ones conventionally used and reported in the scientific literature, are approximately equal to the sample mean plus or minus two standard errors.

The difference between the upper and lower confidence limits is called the **confidence interval** and is sometimes abbreviated as *CI*.

Obviously, researchers will want their confidence intervals to be as narrow as possible. The formula for confidence limits shows that narrowing the confidence interval (for a given level of confidence, such as 95%) requires that the standard error ($\sigma_{\overline{x}}$) be made smaller. Standard error is found by the formula $\sigma_{\overline{x}} = \sigma \div \sqrt{n}$; because σ is a population parameter that the researcher cannot change, the only way the researcher can reduce standard error is by increasing the sample size n. Note that the formula for standard error means that standard error will decrease only in proportion to the *square root* of the sample size; therefore, the width of the confidence interval will also decrease in proportion to the square root of the sample size. In other words, to *halve* the confidence interval, the sample size must be increased *fourfold*.

Precision and accuracy

Precision is the degree to which a figure (such as an estimate of a population mean) is immune to random variation. The width of the confidence interval reflects the precision of the estimate of the population mean—the wider the confidence interval, the less precise the estimate. Because the width of the confidence interval decreases in proportion to the square root of sample size, *precision is proportional to the square root of sample size*. Therefore, to double the precision of an estimate, sample size must be multiplied by four; to triple precision, sample size must be multiplied by nine; and to quadruple precision, sample size must be multiplied by 16, and so on. Increasing the precision of research therefore requires disproportionate increases in sample size—which is why very precise research is expensive and time-consuming.

Precision must be distinguished from **accuracy**, which is the degree to which an estimate is immune from systematic error or bias.

Figure 2-3 illustrates different levels of precision and accuracy in four hypothetical random sampling distributions of means. Each curve shows the result of taking a very large number of samples from the same population and then plotting their means on a frequency distribution. **Precision** is shown by the spread of each curve: as in all frequency distributions, the spread of the distribution around its mean reflects its variability. A very spread-out curve has a high variability and a high standard error and therefore provides an imprecise estimate of the true population mean. **Accuracy** is shown by the distance between the mean of the random sampling distribution of means ($\mu_{\bar{x}}$) and the true population mean (μ).

Distribution A is a very spread-out random sampling distribution of means—as such it provides an **imprecise** estimate of the true population mean. However, its mean does coincide with the true population mean, and therefore it provides an **accurate** estimate of the true population mean. In other words, the estimate that it provides is not biased, but it is subject to considerable random variation. This is the type of result that would occur if the samples were truly random but small.

Distribution B is a narrow distribution, which therefore provides a **precise** estimate of the true population mean. Due to the low standard error, the width of the confidence interval would be narrow. However, its mean lies a long way from the true population mean, so it will provide a **biased** estimate of the true population mean. This is the kind of result that is produced by large but biased (i.e., not truly random) samples.

Distribution C has the worst of both worlds: it is very spread out (having a high standard error) and would therefore provide an **imprecise** estimate of the true population mean. Its mean lies a long way from the true population mean, so its estimate is also **biased**. This would occur if the samples were small and biased.

Distribution D is narrow, and therefore **precise**, and its mean lies at the same point as the true population mean, so it is also **accurate**. This ideal is the kind of distribution that would be obtained from large and truly random samples; therefore, to achieve maximum precision and accuracy in inferential statistics, samples should be large and truly random.

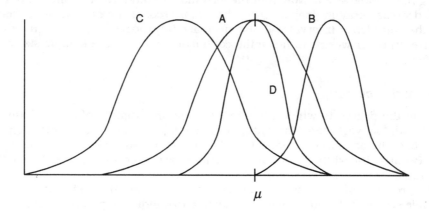

Figure 2-3

Estimating the standard error

So far it has been shown how to determine the probability that a random sample will have a mean of above or below a certain value, and it has been shown how the mean of a sample can be used to estimate the true mean of the population from which it was drawn, with a known degree of precision and confidence. All this has been done by using z scores, which express the number of standard errors by which a sample mean lies above or below the true population mean.

However, because standard error is found from the formula $\sigma_{\overline{x}} - \sigma \div \sqrt{n}$, it requires that σ, the population standard deviation, is known. But in practice σ will not be known; researchers hardly ever know the standard deviation of the population (and if they did, they would probably not need to use inferential statistics anyway).

As a result, standard error cannot be calculated, and therefore z scores cannot be used. Instead, the standard error can be *estimated* using data that are available from the sample alone. The resulting statistic is the **estimated standard error of the mean**, usually called estimated standard error (although, confusingly, it is called standard error in many research articles); it is symbolized by $s_{\overline{x}}$, and it is found by the formula

$$s_{\overline{x}} = \frac{S}{\sqrt{n}}$$

— where S is the sample standard deviation, as defined in Chapter 1.

t scores

The estimated standard error is used to find a statistic that can be used in place of z. This statistic is called t, and in fact t, not z, *must* be used when making inferences about means that are based on *estimates* of population parameters (such as estimated standard error) rather than on the population parameters themselves.

The statistic t (sometimes known as **Student's** t) is calculated similarly to z—but whereas z was expressed in terms of the number of standard errors by which a sample mean lies above or below the population mean, t is expressed in terms of the number of *estimated* standard errors by which the sample mean lies above or below the population mean. The formula for t is therefore

$$t = \frac{\overline{X} - \mu}{s_{\overline{x}}}$$

Compare this formula with the formulas for z on page 21.

Just as tables of z scores state the proportions of the normal distribution that lie above and below any given z score, there are tables of t scores that provide the same information for any given t score. However, there is one difference: whereas the value of z for any given proportion of the distribution is constant (e.g., z values of ± 1.96 *always* delineate the middle 95% of the distribution), the value of t for any given proportion is not constant. The value of t varies from one sample to the next because t is calculated in terms of the estimated standard error ($s_{\overline{x}}$), which in itself varies from sample to sample.

The t distribution varies according to the size of the sample; when the sample size is large ($n > 100$), the values of t and z are similar (because in such large samples, the sample standard deviation provides a good estimate of the standard error). For smaller samples, t and z scores become increasingly different.

Degrees of freedom and *t* tables

Table 2-1 is an abbreviated table of t scores that shows the values of t corresponding to different areas under the normal distribution for various sample sizes. Tables of t values do not show sample size (n) directly; instead, they express sample size in terms of **degrees of freedom** (df). For present purposes, degrees of freedom[2] can be simply defined as being equal to $n - 1$. Therefore, to determine the value of t (such that 95% of the population of t-

statistics based on a sample size of 15 lies between $-t$ and $+t$), one would look in the table for the appropriate value of t for $df = 14$ (14 being equal to $n - 1$); this is sometimes written as t_{14}. Table 2-1 shows that this value is 2.145.

Table 2-1

Area in 2 tails	.100	.050	.010	
Area in 1 tail	.050	.025	.005	
df				
1	6.314	12.706	63.657	
2	2.920	4.303	9.925	
3	2.353	3.182	5.841	
4	2.132	2.776	4.604	
5	2.015	2.571	4.032	
6	1.943	2.447	3.707	
7	1.895	2.365	3.499	
8	1.860	2.306	3.355	
9	1.833	2.262	3.250	
10	1.812	2.228	3.169	
11	1.796	2.201	3.106	
12	1.782	2.179	3.055	
13	1.771	2.160	3.012	
14	1.761	2.145	2.977	
15	1.753	2.131	2.947	
25	1.708	2.060	2.787	
50	1.676	2.009	2.678	
100	1.660	1.984	2.626	
∞	1.645	1.960	2.576	

This table is not a complete listing of t-statistics values. Full tables may be found in most statistics textbooks.

Notice that as n gets large (100 or more), the values of t are very close to the corresponding values of z. As the middle column shows, for a df of 100, 95% of the distribution falls within $t = \pm1.984$; whereas for a df of ∞ this figure is 1.96, which is the same figure as for z (see Table 1-3). In general, the value of t that divides the central 95% of the distribution from the remaining 5% is in the region of 2, just as it is for z; therefore, t_{crit} for a = .05 is generally in the region of 2 (see page 33 for a discussion of t_{crit}). One- and two-tailed tests are discussed on pages 38 and 39.

As an example of the use of t scores, the earlier problem of estimating (with 95% confidence) the true mean resting heart rate of a large population, basing the estimate on the mean heart rate of a random sample of people drawn from this population, can be repeated. This time, the unrealistic assumption that the standard error is known will not be made.

As before, a random sample of 15 people is drawn, and it is found that their mean heart rate ($\overline{X}$) is 74. Assuming that the standard deviation of this sample is 8.2, the estimated standard error, $s_{\overline{X}}$, can be calculated as follows:

$$s_{\overline{X}} = \frac{S}{\sqrt{n-1}}$$

$$= \frac{8.2}{\sqrt{15-1}}$$

$$= \frac{8.2}{3.74}$$

$$= 2.2$$

For a sample consisting of 15 people, the t tables show the appropriate value of t (corresponding to the middle 95% of the distribution) for $df = 14$ (i.e., $n - 1$).

Table 2-1 shows that this value is 2.145. Note that it is not very different from the "ballpark" 95% figure for z, which is 2. The 95% confidence intervals are therefore equal to the sample mean plus or minus t times the estimated standard error (i.e., $\overline{X} \pm t \times s_{\overline{X}}$), which in this example is

$$74 \pm (2.145 \times 2.2) = 69.281 \text{ and } 78.719.$$

The sample mean therefore allows for the estimate that the true mean resting heart rate of this population is 74. One can be 95% confident that it lies between 69.281 and 78.719.

Because the figure for t for 95% confidence intervals is almost invariably going to be in the region of 2 (see Table 2-1), it should be noted that, in general, *one can be 95% confident that the true mean of a population lies within approximately plus or minus two estimated standard errors of the mean of a random sample drawn from the population.*

NOTES

[1] As Table 1-3 shows, the *exact z* scores which correspond to the middle 95% of any normal distribution are in fact ±1.96, not ±2; so the exact limits are $70 \pm (1.96 \times 2) = 66.08$ and 73.92.

[2] Degrees of freedom is properly defined as the number of elements in a distribution that are free to vary when their sum is fixed. In a series of elements with a fixed sum, *all* of the elements are therefore free to vary except for one; hence $df = n - 1$.

EXERCISES

1. What is the name of the standard deviation of the random sampling distribution of means?

2.   What is the formula for the standard deviation of the random sampling distribution of means?

3.   The z score of a single element in a normally distributed population is expressed in terms of the number of standard deviations by which it lies above or below the population mean. In what terms is the z score of a random sample mean expressed?

> For each of the following questions, assume that the population is normally distributed and that the sample is random.

---

4.   If $\overline{X} = 40$, $\mu = 50$, and $\sigma_{\overline{X}} = 5$, what is z?

5.   If $\overline{X} = 100$, $\mu = 85$, and $\sigma_{\overline{X}} = 7.5$, what is z?

6.   If $\sigma = 30$ and $n = 36$, what is $\sigma_{\overline{X}}$?

7.   If $\mu = 100$ and $\sigma_{\overline{X}} = 15$, what is the probability that a random sample drawn from this population will have a mean between 70 and 130?

8.   If $\sigma = 50$ and $n = 25$, what is $\sigma_{\overline{X}}$?

9.   If $\mu = 200$ and $\sigma = 50$, what is the probability that a random sample ($n = 25$) drawn from this population will have a mean above 210 or below 190?

10.   If $\mu = 200$ and $\sigma = 50$, 95% of random sample means ($n = 25$) drawn from this population would lie between what limits?

11.   If μ is unknown, $\sigma = 50$, $\overline{X} = 200$, and $n = 25$, one can be 95% confident that μ lies between what limits?

12.   If μ is unknown, $\sigma = 50$, $\overline{X} = 200$, and $n = 100$, one can be 95% confident that μ lies between what limits?

13.   If μ is unknown, $\sigma = 50$, $\overline{X} = 200$, and $n = 400$, one can be 95% confident that μ lies between what limits?

14.   When $\sigma_{\overline{X}}$ is not known, what is it estimated by?

15. The formula for standard error is $\sigma_{\bar{x}} = \dfrac{\sigma}{\sqrt{n}}$. What is the formula for *estimated* standard error?

16. When standard error is known, z scores are used to determine proportions of the normal distribution. When standard error is not known, what are z scores replaced by?

17. To calculate standard error, σ (population standard deviation) must be known. What is required instead of σ to calculate *estimated* standard error?

18. If $S = 12$ and $n = 10$, what is $s_{\bar{x}}$?

19. If $S = 14$ and $n = 50$, what is $s_{\bar{x}}$?

20. If $S = 3$ and $n = 82$, what is $s_{\bar{x}}$?

21. If $\bar{X} = 46$, $\mu = 50$, and $s_{\bar{x}} = 2$, what is the t value corresponding to the sample mean?

22. If $\bar{X} = 12.4$, $\mu = 10.8$, and $s_{\bar{x}} = 0.8$, what is the t value corresponding to the sample mean?

23. If $n = 12$, what is *df*?

24. If $\bar{X} = 60$, $n = 26$, and $S = 10$, what are the 95% confidence limits for the estimate of μ? (Note that t_{25} for 95% of the distribution is 2.060.)

25. If $\bar{X} = 90$, $n = 63$, $s_{\bar{x}} = 4$, and t for a *df* of 62 and 95% of the distribution is 2.0, what are the 95% confidence limits for the estimate of the population mean?

3

Hypothesis Testing

Chapter 2 showed how a statistic (such as the mean of a sample) can be used to estimate a parameter (such as the mean of a population) with a known degree of confidence. This is an important use of inferential statistics, but a more important use is *hypothesis testing*.

Hypothesis testing may appear complex at first glance, but it involves a series of steps that are straightforward when taken one at a time. In this chapter the following sequence of steps involved in testing a hypothesis about a mean is presented:

1. Stating the null and alternative hypotheses, H_O and H_A

2. Selecting the decision criterion α (or "level of significance")

3. Establishing the critical values

4. Drawing a random sample from the population, and calculating the mean of that sample

5. Calculating the standard deviation (S) and estimated standard error of the sample ($s_{\bar{x}}$)

6. Calculating the value of the test statistic t that corresponds to the mean of the sample (t_{calc})

7. Comparing the calculated value of t with the critical values of t, and then accepting or rejecting the null hypothesis

STEP 1: STATING THE NULL AND ALTERNATIVE HYPOTHESES

Consider the following example. The president of a medical school states that the school's students are a highly intelligent group with an average IQ of 135. This claim constitutes a hypothesis that can be tested; it is called the **null hypothesis**, or **H_O**. It has this name because it is typically the hypothesis that there is no difference between samples or populations being compared (e.g., that a new drug that is being tested produces no change compared with an existing drug). If this hypothesis is rejected as false, then there is an **alternative hypothesis, H_A**, which logically must be accepted. In the case of the school president's claim, the following hypotheses can be stated:

$$\text{Null hypothesis, } H_O : \mu = 135$$

$$\text{Alternative hypothesis, } H_A : \mu \neq 135$$

One way of testing the null hypothesis would be to measure the IQ of every student in the school—in other words, to test the entire population—but this would be an expensive and time-consuming method. A more sensible approach would be to draw a random sample of students, find their mean IQ, and then draw inferences from this sample mean.

STEP 2: SELECTING THE DECISION CRITERION α

If the null hypothesis were correct, would the mean IQ of the random sample of students be expected to be exactly 135? No, of course not; as shown in Chapter 2, there will always be a sampling error that will cause the mean IQ of the sample to deviate somewhat from the mean IQ of the population (135). For example, if the mean IQ of the sample were 134, it could reasonably be concluded that the null hypothesis had not been contradicted, because chance sampling error could easily permit this sample to have been drawn from a population with a mean of 135. To reach a conclusion about the null hypothesis, it must therefore be decided *at what point is the difference between the sample mean and 135 not due to chance* but due to the fact that the population mean is *not* really 135, as the null hypothesis claims?

This point must be set before the sample is drawn and the data collected. Instead of setting it in terms of the actual IQ score, it is set in terms of probability. The probability level at which it is decided that the null hypothesis is incorrect constitutes a **criterion**, or significance level, known as α (alpha). As the random sampling distribution of means shows, it is unlikely that a random sample will have a mean that is *very* different from the true population mean—the sample mean is unlikely to lie very far toward either of the two tails of the random sampling distribution of means. If the sample mean *does* lie very far toward one of the tails of this distribution, it must arouse suspicion that the sample was *not* drawn from the population specified in the null hypothesis. In other words, the greater the difference between the sample mean and the hypothesized population mean, the less probable it is that the sample really does come from a population with the hypothesized mean; and when this probability is very low, it can be concluded that the null hypothesis is incorrect.

How low does this probability need to be for the null hypothesis to be rejected as incorrect? It is conventional to state that the null hypothesis will be rejected if the probability of having obtained the sample mean from the hypothesized population is less than or equal to .05; therefore, the conventional level of α is .05. Conversely, if the probability of obtaining the sample mean is greater than .05, the null hypothesis will be accepted as correct. Although α may be set lower than the conventional .05 (for reasons which will be shown later), it cannot normally be set any higher than this.

STEP 3: ESTABLISHING THE CRITICAL VALUES

Chapter 2 showed that if a very large number of random samples are taken from any population, their means form a normal distribution—the random sampling distribution of means—which has a mean ($\mu_{\bar{x}}$) equal to the population mean (μ). It has also been shown that one can state what random sample means are so high or so low that they would occur in only 5% or fewer of all possible random samples. Therefore, the problem of testing this null hypothesis about the students' mean IQ involves establishing which random sample means would be so high or so low that they would occur in only 5% (or fewer) of all random samples that could be drawn from a population with a mean of 135.

If the obtained sample mean falls inside the range within which 95% of random sample means would be expected to fall, the null hypothesis is accepted. This range is therefore called the **area of acceptance**. But if the sample mean falls outside this range, in the

area of rejection, the null hypothesis is rejected, and the alternative hypothesis must be accepted.

The limits of this range are called the **critical values**, which are established by referring to a table of t scores. The sample size in this example is 10; therefore, there are $(n - 1) = 9$ degrees of freedom. The table of t scores (Table 2-1) shows that when $df = 9$, the value of t that divides the 95% (.95) area of acceptance from the two 2.5% (.025) areas of rejection is ±2.262. These are therefore the critical values, which can be written $t_{crit} = ±2.262$.

Figure 3-1 shows the random sampling distribution of means for the hypothesized population in which $\mu = 135$, together with the areas of rejection and acceptance delimited by the critical values of t just established. The hypothesized population mean is sometimes written μ_{hyp}.

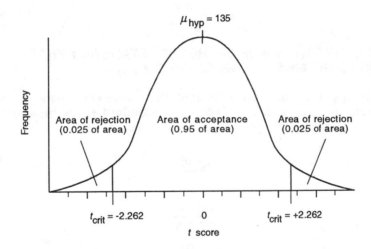

Figure 3-1

Having established the null and alternative hypotheses, the criterion that will determine when the null hypothesis will be accepted or rejected, and the critical values of t associated with this criterion, the random sample of students can now be drawn from the population. Then, the t score (t_{calc}) associated with the mean IQ of this sample can be calculated and compared with the critical values of t. This constitutes a **t-test**—a commonly used procedure in medical research.

STEP 4: DRAWING A RANDOM SAMPLE FROM THE POPULATION AND CALCULATING THE MEAN OF THAT SAMPLE

The random sample of 10 students is drawn; their IQs turn out to be as follows:

$$115...140...133...125...120...126...136...124...132...129$$

The mean ($\overline{X}$) of this sample of ten IQs is 128.

STEP 5: CALCULATING THE STANDARD DEVIATION (*S*) AND ESTIMATED STANDARD ERROR OF THE SAMPLE ($s_{\overline{X}}$)

To calculate the *t* score corresponding to the sample mean, the estimated standard error must first be found. This is done in the usual way (as explained in Chapter 2): the standard deviation (*S*) of this sample is calculated, and is found to be 7.155; then, the estimated standard error ($s_{\overline{X}}$) is calculated as follows:

$$s_{\overline{X}} = \frac{S}{\sqrt{n-1}}$$

$$= \frac{7.155}{\sqrt{10-1}}$$

$$= 2.385$$

STEP 6: CALCULATING THE VALUE OF THE TEST STATISTIC *t* THAT CORRESPONDS TO THE MEAN OF THE SAMPLE (t_{CALC})

Now that the standard error has been estimated, the *t* score corresponding to the sample mean can be found; it is the number of estimated standard errors by which the sample mean lies above or below the hypothesized population mean:

$$t = \frac{\overline{X} - \mu_{hyp}}{s_{\overline{X}}}$$

$$= \frac{128 - 135}{2.385}$$

$$= -2.935$$

STEP 7: COMPARING THE CALCULATED VALUE OF *t* WITH THE CRITICAL VALUES OF *t*, AND THEN ACCEPTING OR REJECTING THE NULL HYPOTHESIS

If the calculated value of *t* corresponding to the sample mean falls at or beyond either of the critical values, it falls within one of the two areas of rejection. Figure 3-2 shows that the *t* score in this example does, in fact, fall within the lower area of rejection. Therefore, the null hypothesis is rejected and the alternative hypothesis is accepted, because the sample mean is so different from the hypothesized population mean that the probability of having obtained it if the null hypothesis were true is only .05 (or less). In other words, the probability that this sample could have come from a population with a mean of 135 is so low that it can be concluded that the population mean is not 135. It can be said that the difference between the sample mean and the hypothesized population mean is **statistically significant**, and that the null hypothesis has been rejected at the .05 level. This would typically be reported as follows: "The hypothesis that the mean IQ of the population is 135 was rejected, *t* = -2.935, *df* = 9, *p* ≤ .05."

If, on the other hand, the calculated value of *t* corresponding to the sample mean had fallen *between* the two critical values, in the area of acceptance, the null hypothesis would have to be accepted instead, and it could be stated that the difference between the sample mean and the hypothesized population mean failed to reach statistical significance.

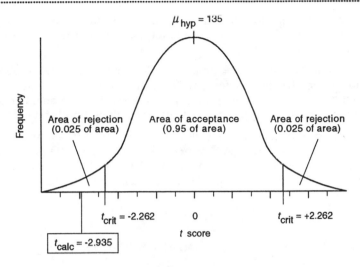

Figure 3-2

In some situations the sequence of steps just followed can be done using z scores instead of t scores—this is called a **z-test**. This is possible if the population standard deviation is known, which allows the standard error itself (rather than the estimated error) to be found in step 6; or when the sample is sufficiently large ($n \geq 100$) for the sample standard deviation to provide a reliable estimate of the standard error. Although there are situations in which a t-test can be used but a z-test cannot, there are no situations in which a z-test can be used but a t-test cannot—so t-tests are the more important and widely used of the two.

THE MEANING OF STATISTICAL SIGNIFICANCE

To report that a result is statistically significant at a certain level p, with a statement such as "significant at $p \leq .05$," merely means that the result was unlikely to have occurred by chance—specifically, that the likelihood of the result having occurred by chance is .05 or less. But this does *not* necessarily mean that the result is *substantively* significant, i.e., that it is significant in the everyday meaning of the word—that it is important, noteworthy, or meaningful.

For example, if the mean IQ of the sample of students was found to be 134, it is possible (if the sample were large enough) that this mean could fall in the area of rejection; the null hypothesis that the mean IQ of the population is 135 could be rejected. But this would scarcely be an important or noteworthy disproof of the school president's claim.[1]

Similarly, a study comparing the efficacy of two antihypertensive drugs might conclude that one drug produced a statistically significant lower mean blood pressure than the other; but if the difference were only 1 mm Hg, this would not be a *substantively* significant finding, and would not necessarily cause physicians to prescribe this drug rather than the other.

TYPE I AND TYPE II ERRORS

If an investigator reports that a result is significant by stating that $p \leq .05$, this means that the investigator is 95% sure that the result was not obtained by chance. It also means that there is still a 5% probability that the result *could* have been obtained by chance. So although the investigator is rejecting the null hypothesis, it may, nevertheless, still be true: there remains a 5% chance that the data *did*, in fact, come from the population specified by the null hypothesis.[2]

To reject a null hypothesis when it is true is to make a **type I** or **"false negative" error**, which means a false negative conclusion has been drawn about the null hypothesis. The value of α (or p) is in fact the probability that a type I error is being made; because this value corresponds to the criterion α, a type I error is also known as an **alpha error**.

The opposite kind of error, accepting the null hypothesis when it is actually false (drawing a **"false positive"** conclusion) is a **type II** or **beta error**. Whereas the probability of making a type I error is α, the probability of making a type II error is β. Table 3-1 shows the four possible types of decisions that can be made on the basis of statistical tests.

Table 3-1

ACTUAL SITUATION

		H_o true	H_o false
T E S T R E S U L T	H_o accepted	Correct	Type II error (β)
	H_o rejected	Type I error (α)	Correct

The choice of an appropriate level for the criterion α therefore depends on the relative consequences of making a type I or a type II error. For example, if a study is expensive and time-consuming (and is therefore unlikely to be repeated), while having important practical implications, the researchers may wish to establish a more stringent level of α (such as .01, .005, or even .001) to be more than 95% sure that their conclusions are correct. This was done in the multimillion dollar Lipid Research Clinics Coronary Primary Prevention Trial, whose planners stated that

> since the time, magnitude, and costs of this study make it unlikely that it could ever be repeated, it was essential that any observed benefit of total cholesterol lowering was a real one. Therefore, α was set to .01 rather than the usual .05.

> (Lipid Research Clinics Program, 1979)

Although the criterion to be selected need not be .05, by convention it cannot be any higher. Results that do not quite reach the .05 level of probability are sometimes reported to "approach significance" or to "show statistically significant trends."

Many researchers do not state a predetermined criterion or report their results in terms of one; instead, they report the actual probability of the obtained result having occurred by chance if the null hypothesis were true (e.g., "$p \leq .015$"). In these cases, the p value is more an "index of rarity" than a true decision criterion. The researchers are showing how unlikely it is that a type I error has been made, even though they would have still rejected the null hypothesis if the outcome were only significant at the .05 level.

POWER OF STATISTICAL TESTS

Although it is possible to guard against a type I error simply by using a more stringent (lower) level of α, preventing a type II error is not so easy. Because a type II error involves accepting a false null hypothesis, the ability of a statistical test to avoid a type II error depends on its ability to detect a null hypothesis that is false. This ability is called the **power** of the test, and it is equal to $1 - \beta$. It is the probability that a false null hypothesis will be rejected. Conventionally, a study is required to have a power of 0.8 to be acceptable—in other words, it is generally judged that a study that has a less than 80% chance of detecting a false null hypothesis is unacceptable.

Calculating β, thereby determining the power of a test, is complex. But it is clear that a test's power, or ability to detect a false null hypothesis, will increase as:

- α increases, e.g., from .01 to .05. This will make the critical values of t less extreme, thus increasing the size of the areas of rejection and making rejection of the null hypothesis more likely. There will always be a trade-off between type I and type II errors: increasing α reduces the chance of a type II error, but at the same time it increases the chance of a type I error.

- the size of the difference between the sample mean and the hypothesized population mean increases (this is known as the **effect size**). In the preceding example, a difference between a hypothesized population mean IQ of 135 and a sample mean IQ of 100 would be detected much more easily (and hence the null hypothesis would be rejected more easily) than a difference between a hypothesized IQ of 135 and a sample mean IQ of 128. The larger the difference, the more extreme the calculated value of t.

- sampling error decreases. A lower sampling error means that the sample standard deviation (S) is reduced, which will cause the estimated standard error ($s_{\bar{x}}$) to be lower. Because t is calculated in terms of estimated standard errors, this will make the calculated value of t more extreme (whether in a positive or negative direction), increasing the likelihood that it falls in one of the areas of rejection.

- the sample size (n) increases; this reduces the estimated standard error ($s_{\bar{x}}$), thereby increasing the calculated value of t. Therefore, a large-scale study is more likely to detect a false null hypothesis (particularly if the effect size is small) than is a small-scale study. For example, if a coin is tossed 1000 times resulting in 600 heads and 400 tails, one is much more able to reject the null hypothesis that the coin is a fair one than if the coin is tossed 10 times and six heads and four tails are obtained.

Increasing the sample size is the most practical and important way of increasing the power of a statistical test. Researchers who dispute the findings of a study in which the null hypothesis is accepted, claiming that it is an example of a type II error, may argue that the study's sample was too small to detect a real difference or effect. Under such circumstances they may choose to replicate the study, using a larger sample to improve the likelihood of getting statistically significant results that allow them to reject the null hypothesis.

In practice, researchers will attempt to predict the likely effect size before they begin a study, so that they can use a sample size large enough to detect it. They do not simply guess, for instance, that 50 or 500 patients will be needed to test a new drug. Ideally, all studies that report acceptance of the null hypothesis should also report the power of the test used, so that the probability of a type II error is made clear.

DIRECTIONAL HYPOTHESES

So far, the example of hypothesis testing has used a **nondirectional** alternative hypothesis, which merely stated that the population mean is *not* equal to 135, but it did not specify whether the population mean is above or below this figure. This was appropriate because the school's president claimed that the students' mean IQ was 135. His claim (which constitutes the null hypothesis) could legitimately be rejected if the sample mean IQ turned out to be significantly above *or* below 135. Therefore, as Figure 3-2 showed, there were *two* areas of rejection, one above μ_{hyp} and one below.

But what if the school's president had instead claimed that the students' average IQ was *at least* 135? This claim could only be rejected if the sample mean IQ turned out to be significantly *lower* than 135. The null hypothesis is now $\mu \geq 135$, and the alternative hypothesis must now be $\mu < 135$. The alternative hypothesis is now a **directional** one, which specifies that the population mean lies in a *particular direction* with respect to the null hypothesis.

In this kind of situation, there are no longer two areas of rejection on the random sampling distribution of means. As Figure 3-3 shows, there is now only one. If α remains at .05, the area of acceptance (the area in which 95% of the means of possible samples drawn from the hypothesized population lie) now extends down from the very top end of the distribution, leaving just *one* area of rejection—the bottom 5% of the curve. The area of rejection now lies in only one tail of the distribution, rather than in both tails.

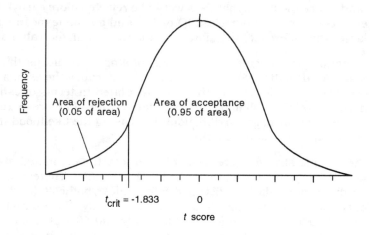

Figure 3-3

The steps involved in conducting a *t*-test of this directional null hypothesis are exactly the same as before, except that the critical value of *t* is now different. The critical value now divides the bottom 5% tail of the distribution from the upper 95%, instead of dividing the middle 95% from two tails of 2.5% each. The appropriate column of Table 2-1 shows that the new critical value of *t* (for the same *df* of 9) is -1.833, rather than the previous value of ±2.262.

As Figure 3-3 shows, this new critical value is associated with only one tail of the distribution. Using this value therefore involves performing a **one-tailed** statistical test, due to the fact that the alternative hypothesis is directional; previously, when the alternative hypothesis was nondirectional, the test performed was a **two-tailed** test.

Notice that the critical value of *t* is less extreme for the one-tailed test (-1.833) than for the two-tailed test (±2.262). Consequently, when a one-tailed test is used, a less extreme sample mean is able to exceed the critical value and fall within the area of rejection, leading to rejection of the null hypothesis. As a result of this, one-tailed tests are more powerful than two-tailed tests.

For example, if the mean IQ of the sample of 10 students were 130 (instead of 128), with the same standard deviation (7.155) and the same estimated standard error (2.385) as before, the value of *t* corresponding to this mean would be

$$\frac{130 - 135}{2.385} = -2.096$$

This score falls within the area of acceptance for a two-tailed test, but it falls within the area of rejection for a one-tailed test, as shown in Figure 3-3. The president's claim could therefore potentially be supported *or* rejected, depending on how it is interpreted and which test is consequently performed.

Under some circumstances a researcher who wishes to reject the null hypothesis may find that by using a one-tailed rather than a two-tailed test, a previously nonsignificant result may become a statistically significant one. For this reason it is important that one-tailed tests are only performed under the correct conditions. The decision to use a one-tailed test must depend on *the nature of the hypothesis being tested, and should therefore be decided at the outset of the research*, rather than being decided afterward according to how the results turn out.

One-tailed tests can only be used when there is a directional alternative hypothesis. This means that they may not be used unless results in only one direction are of interest, and the possibility of the results being in the opposite direction is of no interest or consequence to the researcher.

When testing a new drug, the normal null hypothesis is that the drug has no effect, so it will be rejected if the drug turns out to have an effect too great to be due to chance, irrespective of whether the effect is a positive one or a negative one. Although the researcher *expects* the drug to produce an improvement in patients' symptoms, this expectation does not permit the use of a directional alternative hypothesis. The researcher can do this only if it is of no interest or consequence if the drug actually makes patients worse—a claim that can almost never be made legitimately in biomedical research.

It is generally appropriate to use a directional alternative hypothesis (and hence a one-tailed test) only in public health work—such as when a researcher wants to establish that a product does not fall below a particular minimum standard of purity, but is not concerned with discovering by what margin it exceeds the standard as long as the standard is being met.

If the law requires that bottled drinking water contain no more than eight parts per million (ppm) of lead, a public health official will wish to test the null hypothesis that the mean level of lead in a certain brand of water is 8 ppm or less. The alternative hypothesis is therefore that the mean level of lead is *more than* 8 ppm; as this is a directional alternative hypothesis, a one-tailed test can be used. If the researcher examines a random sample of 20 bottles of the water, and as a result accepts the null hypothesis, the water may be sold. It makes no practical difference whether the level of lead is 8 ppm, 5 ppm, 2 ppm, or even less—the consequences are always the same: the null hypothesis is always accepted, and the water may be sold. The official is *only* interested if the sample mean differs from the hypothesized population mean in one specific direction—i.e., if the sample mean turns out to be significantly *greater* than 8 ppm. If it turns out to be significantly *less* than 8 ppm, the consequences are no different from it being *equal* to 8 ppm.

TESTING FOR DIFFERENCES BETWEEN GROUPS

It has been shown how a *t*-test can be used to test a hypothesis about a single mean. However, biomedical research is often more complex than this: researchers commonly want to compare *two* means, such as the mean effects of two different drugs or the mean survival times of patients receiving two different treatments.

A slightly more complex version of the *t*-test can be used to test for a significant difference between two means. The null hypothesis is that the two groups were drawn from populations with the same mean—in other words, that the two samples were in effect drawn from the same population, and that there is no difference between them. The alternative hypothesis is that the two population means are different:

$$H_0 : \mu_A = \mu_B$$
$$H_A : \mu_A \neq \mu_B$$

Many research problems involve comparing *more than two groups*; for example, comparing the treatment outcomes of three groups of depressed patients—one group taking a placebo, another a tricyclic antidepressant, the third a monoamine oxidase inhibitor (MAOI) antidepressant. If each group consists of male and female patients, the researcher may also want to make comparisons between the sexes, giving a total of six groups: three different treatment groups, with two sexes within each group. Therefore, the null hypothesis is

$$H_0 : \mu_A = \mu_B = \mu_C = \mu_D = \mu_E = \mu_F$$

In theory, this hypothesis could be tested by multiple *t*-tests, comparing A with B, A with C, A with D, A with E, A with F, B with C, and so on. But this method has some important disadvantages:

- It is time-consuming because it involves performing 15 separate *t*-tests.

- The power of each test is relatively low because each test uses the elements in only two groups, and not the sample as a whole.

- With an α of .05, each test has a .05 chance of producing a type I error; with 15 tests, the probability of at least one of them producing a type I error is unacceptably high.

- The 15 tests will produce 15 separate specific answers (e.g., "men taking an MAOI responded better than women taking a placebo").

It would be more convenient if an *overall* answer were first obtained to see if there were *any* statistically significant differences in the data. Then broad questions like "Is there a significant difference between the three treatments?" could be answered before finally looking for significant differences between subgroups. This is especially true if the researcher has some general expectations (e.g., that depressed men have a better prognosis than women) but has no specific expectations about differences between particular subgroups.

Fortunately, there is a technique that overcomes these problems: **analysis of variance** (or **ANOVA**). Whereas a t-test is appropriate for making just one comparison (between two sample means, or between a sample mean and a hypothesized population mean), when more than one comparison is being made (i.e., when means of more than two groups are being compared), ANOVA is the appropriate technique. Consequently, ANOVA is one of the most commonly used statistical techniques.

ANALYSIS OF VARIANCE

The actual computation of ANOVA is complex and is not required for the USMLE. However, the logic behind it is important. In any set of experimental results, such as the results of the study of antidepressant drugs in the previous section, there will be some variability. The total variability in the results is made up of two components:

1. The variability resulting from the known different factors affecting the different groups: the use of the placebo, the tricyclic antidepressant, the MAOI antidepressant, and the gender of the patient. Each of these factors may affect the results and therefore contribute to the total variability in the results. This is called the **between-group** variance—it is due to the differences *between* the groups.

2. The ordinary random variability that is to be expected in any set of data, caused by sampling error, individual differences between the patients, and so on. This is the **within-group** variance, because it occurs *within* each of the groups.

The essential question is this: can a significant proportion of the overall variability found in the results be attributed to the known differences between the groups or not? ANOVA breaks the total variability down into the preceding two components and compares the variance *between* the different groups with the variance *within* the groups. If the variance between the different groups is large compared with the random fluctuations found within the groups, then it must be due to some difference between the groups above and beyond the random fluctuations. If the experiment has been performed correctly, this difference must be due (in this example) to the gender of the patients or the treatments that they were given, because there is no other non-random difference between the groups.

The F-ratio

ANOVA compares the variance between the groups with the variance within the groups by means of a simple ratio, which is called the **F-ratio**:

$$F = \frac{\text{variance between groups}}{\text{variance within groups}}$$

The resulting F statistic (F_{calc}) is then compared with the critical value of F (F_{crit}), obtained from F tables in much the same way as was done with t. Like t, if the calculated value exceeds the critical value for the appropriate level of α, the null hypothesis will be rejected. An **F-test** is therefore a test of the *ratio of variances*.

F-tests can also be used on their own, independently of the ANOVA technique, to test hypotheses about variances. For example, two different vaccines A and B may produce the same mean antibody concentration, but one vaccine may produce levels that are more variable than the other. An F-test would be used to establish if the difference in their variances is merely due to chance or is statistically significant. The null hypothesis would be $\sigma^2_A = \sigma^2_B$.

In ANOVA, the F-test is used to establish whether a statistically significant difference exists in the data being tested. It will show if there are significant sources of variability in the data above and beyond the expected random variability.

If the various experimental groups differ in terms of only one factor at a time—such as the type of drug being used—a **one-way** ANOVA is used. If the variance between groups is sufficiently large, compared with the variance within groups, for the F-ratio to reach significance, it would then be known that drug type was a significant source of variation in the results.

On the other hand, if the various groups differ in terms of two factors at a time, then a **two-way** ANOVA is performed. This is what would be required if the groups differ not only in terms of drug type but also in terms of gender. This ANOVA will show not only if there are significant sources of variability in the results—it will also show if this variability is attributable to one factor (drug type), to the other factor (gender), or to the two factors in combination with each other.

In more complex experiments, the various groups may differ in terms of three factors simultaneously, requiring a three-way ANOVA; if they differ in terms of four factors, then a four-way ANOVA is used, and so on. Any type of ANOVA above a one-way procedure is also known as a **multifactorial** ANOVA.

Once the existence of statistically significant effects has been established by ANOVA, **post hoc tests** of various kinds can be used to look for statistically significant differences between any specific pair of groups; e.g., to find if the MAOI group differs from the placebo group, if the tricyclic group differs from the placebo group, or if the MAOI and tricyclic groups differ from each other. These *post hoc* tests are also known as **multiple comparison** techniques, because they are used to make multiple comparisons between pairs of groups. Several different techniques of this kind are widely used, including the **Scheffé**, **Tukey**, **Newman-Keuls**, and **Duncan** tests.

If a single factor is found to have a significant effect, it is called a **main effect**. If a combination of factors has a significant effect, this is called an **interaction effect**. Interaction effects occur when the effect of two factors together differs from the sum of the individual effects of each alone.

Graphical presentations of ANOVA data

Main and interaction effects are more easily understood visually. In the example of the study of the effects of MAOIs, tricyclics, and placebos on male and female depressed patients, assume that the results show that the best outcomes were among the patients who took the tricyclics, followed by those who took the MAOIs, and that the worst outcomes were among the patients who took the placebo; and also assume that there are no differences attributable to the gender of the patients.

Figure 3-4 shows these results: provided the differences are large enough to reach statistical significance, a two-way ANOVA would allow the conclusion that there is a main effect due to drug type, that there is no effect due to patient gender, and that there is no effect due to an interaction between drug type and patient gender.

Now assume that in addition to these drug effects, female patients have better outcomes than male patients in each of the three treatment groups. Figure 3-5 illustrates this result;

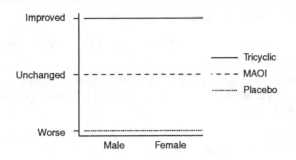

Figure 3-4

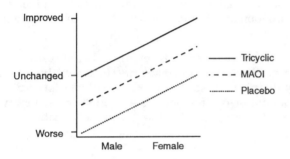

Figure 3-5

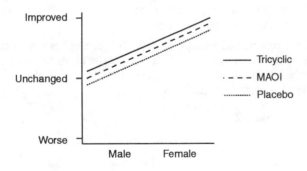

Figure 3-6

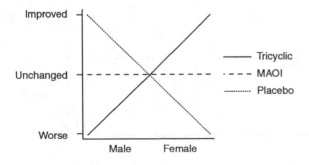

Figure 3-7

here there is a main effect of drug, a main effect of gender, and no interaction effect.

Now assume instead that the three different treatments all produced identical results, and yet the female patients still exhibited better outcomes within each of these treatment groups. Figure 3-6 shows this result; here there is a main effect of gender but no main effect of drug and no interaction effect.

Figure 3-7 shows a fourth possible kind of result: the three treatment groups produce identical *mean* effects when both sexes are considered together; and the male and female patient groups have identical *mean* outcomes when all three drugs are considered together; but there are, in fact, strong effects associated with particular *combinations* of gender and drug type.

In this situation, although there is no main effect of drug and no main effect of gender, there is, nevertheless, a strong *interaction effect* of drug and gender (this would usually be reported as "a strong drug × gender interaction"). Here, the sum of the individual effects of each drug is approximately zero. The *overall* mean effect of each drug is to produce an unchanged outcome; similarly, the sum of the individual effects for either sex is approximately zero; but the effects of particular combinations of drug and patient gender are very different.

Note that when the lines representing different groups on graphs of this kind are parallel, there are no interactions. When they are not parallel, an interaction effect is present (although it is not necessarily a strong or statistically significant one). Interaction effects reach maximum strength when the lines are at right angles to each other.

NONPARAMETRIC AND DISTRIBUTION-FREE TESTS

The previous sections have dealt with t-, z-, and F-tests, which test hypotheses about means or variances. These tests share three common features:

1. Their hypotheses refer to *population parameters:* the population mean (in the case of t- and z-tests) or the population variance (in the case of F-tests). For this reason such tests are called **parametric** tests.

2. Their hypotheses concern *interval* or *ratio* scale data, such as weight, blood pressure, IQ, per capita income, measures of clinical improvement, and so on.

3. They make certain assumptions about the distribution of the data of interest in the population—principally, that the population data are normally distributed. (As was shown earlier, the central limit theorem allows this assumption to be made, even when little is known about the population distribution, provided that random samples of sufficient size are used.)

Other statistical techniques exist that do not share these features: they do not test hypotheses concerning parameters, and hence are known as **nonparametric** tests; they do not assume that the population is normally distributed, so they are also called **distribution-free** tests; and they are used to test nominal or ordinal scale data. Such tests, however, have the disadvantage that they are generally *less powerful* than parametric tests.

Chi-square

The most important nonparametric test is the **chi-square** (χ^2) test, which is used for testing hypotheses about *nominal scale* data. It is basically a test of *proportions:* the question being asked is whether the proportions of observations falling in different categories differ significantly from the proportions that would be expected by chance.

For example, in tossing a coin 100 times, one would expect 50% (or 50) of the tosses to fall in the category of heads and 50 to fall in the category of tails. If the result is 59 heads and 41 tails, chi-square would show whether this difference in proportion is too large to be expected by chance— i.e., whether it is statistically significant.

Table 3-2

	School A	School B	School C	
Number Passing	49	112	26	Total 187
Number Rejected	12	37	8	Total 57
Total	61	149	34	

As with other tests, chi-square involves calculating the test statistic (χ^2_{calc}) according to a standard formula and comparing it with the critical value (appropriate for the level of α selected) shown in the published chi-square tables. These tables can be found in most statistics textbooks.

Chi-square is also used in more complicated analyses involving nominal scale data. For example, a study might compare the USMLE pass rates of candidates from three different medical schools shown in Table 3-2. This kind of table is a **contingency table**; it expresses the idea that one variable (such as passing or failing the examination) may be contingent on the other (such as which medical school one attended). Data to be tested using chi-square are typically presented in the form of such a table.

The question that chi-square can answer is this: is there a relationship between which school the student attended and passing or failing the exam? A simple formula allows the value of chi-square to be calculated; if it exceeds the critical value, the null hypothesis (that there is no relationship) is rejected.

NOTES

[1] In fact, virtually *any* null hypothesis can be rejected if the sample is sufficiently large, because there will almost always be some trivial difference between the hypothesized mean and the sample mean (Kupfersmid, 1988). Studies using extremely large samples are therefore at risk of producing findings that are statistically significant but substantively insignificant.

[2] Many statistics textbooks and researchers erroneously take this to mean that there is therefore a 5% chance that the null hypothesis is in fact still true, although it is being rejected. The *p* or α value is the probability that the data could have come from the population specified by the null hypothesis, *not* the other way around (Hill, 1990).

EXERCISES

A medical student believes that interns get less sleep than the general population of young adults. He decides to test this hypothesis by taking a random sample of 10 interns on a randomly selected day, and asking them how many hours they slept the previous night. He then compares their mean number of hours of sleep with that of the general population of young adults, which he assumes to be 8 hours per night.

1. What is the null hypothesis H_0?

2. What is the alternative hypothesis H_A?

3. Under what circumstances would a directional alternative hypothesis, and therefore a one-tailed test, be used?

4. The 10 interns' hours of sleep are: 2, 4, 6, 6, 6, 7, 7, 8, 10, and 14. $\Sigma X = 70$; what is the sample mean $\overline{X}$?

5. $\Sigma x^2 = 83$; what is the sample variance S^2?

6.   If $\sqrt{8.3} = 2.88$, what is the approximate value of the estimated standard error $s_{\bar{x}}$?

7.   What is the approximate value of t_{calc}?

8.   If t_{crit} for $df = 9$ and $\alpha = .05$ is ± 2.262, is the null hypothesis accepted or rejected?

9.   How might the power of this statistical test be most readily improved?

10.   There is no real reason to suppose that interns' hours of sleep are normally distributed. Does this mean that a t-test cannot be used?

11.   If this test was not powerful enough to detect a real difference between the interns' mean number of hours of sleep and that of the null hypothesis, what type of error is being made here?

12.   What is the best estimate of the mean number of hours of sleep of the population of all interns?

13.   What are the approximate 95% confidence limits of this estimate?

4

Correlational Techniques

Biomedical research often seeks to establish if there is a relationship between two variables; for example, is there a relationship between people's salt intake and their blood pressure, or between the number of cigarettes they smoke and their life expectancy? The methods used to do this are **correlational** techniques, which focus on the "co-relatedness" of the two variables. There are two basic kinds of correlational technique:

1. **Correlation** itself, which is used to establish and quantify the *strength* and *direction* of the relationship between two variables.

2. **Regression**, which is used to express the *functional relationship* between two variables, so that the value of one variable can be *predicted* from knowledge of the other.

CORRELATION

A correlation simply expresses the strength and direction of the relationship between two variables in terms of a **correlation coefficient**, signified by r. Values of r vary from -1 to +1; the strength of the relationship is indicated by the size of the coefficient, whereas its direction is indicated by the sign.

A plus sign means that there is a **positive correlation** between the two variables—high values of one variable (such as salt intake) are associated with high values of the other variable (such as blood pressure). A minus sign means that there is a **negative correlation** between the two variables—high values of one variable (such as cigarette consumption) are associated with low values of the other (such as life expectancy).

If there is a "perfect" linear relationship between the two variables, so that it is possible to know the exact value of one variable from knowledge of the other variable, the correlation coefficient (r) will be exactly plus or minus 1.00. If there is absolutely no relationship between the two variables, so that it is impossible to know anything about one variable on the basis of knowledge of the other variable, then the coefficient will be zero. Coefficients beyond ±0.5 are typically regarded as strong, whereas coefficients between zero and ±0.5 are usually regarded as weak.

Scattergrams and bivariate distributions

The relationship between two variables being correlated forms a **bivariate distribution**, which is commonly presented graphically in the form of a **scattergram**. The first variable (salt intake, cigarette consumption) is usually plotted on the horizontal (X) axis, whereas the second variable (blood pressure, life expectancy) is plotted on the vertical (Y) axis. Each plotted data point represents one observation of a pair of values, such as one patient's salt intake and blood pressure, so the number of plotted points is equal to the sample size n. Figure 4-1 shows four different scattergrams.

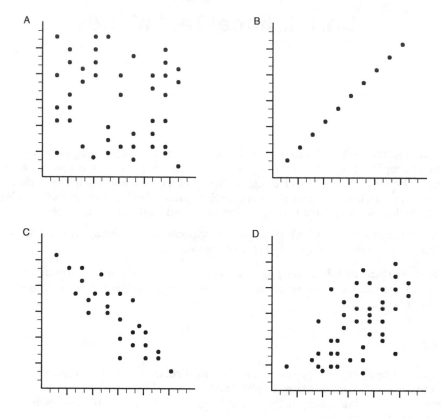

Figure 4-1

Determining a correlation coefficient involves mathematically finding the straight "line of best fit" that fits the plotted data points most closely. The relationship between the appearance of the scattergram and the correlation coefficient can therefore be understood by imagining how well such a line could be drawn to fit the plotted points. In Figure 4-1(A), for example, it is not possible to draw any straight line that would fit the plotted points *at all*; therefore, the correlation coefficient is zero. In Figure 4-1(B), a straight line would fit the plotted points perfectly—so the correlation coefficient is 1.00. Figure 4-1(C) shows a strong negative correlation, whereas Figure 4-1(D) shows a weak positive correlation.

Types of correlation coefficient

The two most commonly used correlation coefficients are the **Pearson product-moment correlation**, which is used for *interval* or *ratio* scale data, and the **Spearman rank-order correlation**, which is used for *ordinal* scale data. The latter is sometimes symbolized by the letter ρ (rho). Pearson's r would therefore be used (for example) to express the association between salt intake and blood pressure (which are both ratio scale data), whereas Spearman's ρ would be used to express the association between birth order and class position at school (which are both ordinal scale data).

Both these correlational techniques are **linear**: they evaluate the strength of a "straight line" relationship between the two variables. So if there is a very strong **nonlinear** relationship between two variables, the Pearson or Spearman correlation coefficient will be an underestimate of the true strength of the relationship.

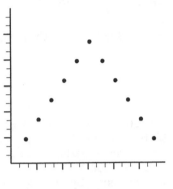

Figure 4-2

Figure 4-2 illustrates such a situation: a drug has a strong effect at medium dosage levels, but very weak effects at very high or very low doses. Because the relationship between dose and effect is so nonlinear, the Pearson r would be very low, even though there is actually a very strong relationship between the two variables. Visual inspection of scattergrams is therefore invaluable in identifying relationships of this sort. More advanced nonlinear correlational techniques can be used to quantify correlations of this kind.

Coefficient of determination

Once a correlation coefficient has been determined, the **coefficient of determination** can be calculated by *squaring the value of r*. The coefficient of determination, symbolized by r^2, expresses the proportion of the variance in one variable that is accounted for, or "explained," by the variance in the other variable. So if a study finds a correlation (r) of .40 between salt intake and blood pressure, it could be concluded that $.40 \times .40 = .16$, or 16% of the variance in blood pressure in this study is accounted for by variance in salt intake.

Note that a correlation between two variables *does NOT demonstrate a causal relationship* between the two variables, no matter how strong it is. Correlation is merely a measure of the variables' statistical association, not of their causal relationship. *Inferring a causal relationship between two variables on the basis of a correlation is a common and fundamental error.*

Furthermore, the fact that a correlation is present between two variables in a sample does not necessarily mean that the correlation actually exists in the population. When a correlation has been found between two variables in a sample, the researcher will normally wish to test the null hypothesis that there is no correlation between the two variables (i.e., that $r = 0$) in the population. This is done with a special form of t-test.

REGRESSION

If two variables are highly correlated, it then becomes possible to *predict* the value of the dependent variable from the value of the independent variable by using **regression** techniques. In the most basic form of this technique, **simple linear regression**, the value of one variable (X) is used to predict the value of the other variable (Y) by means of a simple linear mathematical function, the **regression equation**, which quantifies the straight-line relationship between the two variables. This straight line, or **regression line**, is actually the same "line of best fit" to the scattergram as that used in calculating the correlation coefficient.

The simple linear regression equation takes the same form as the equation for any straight line:

$$\text{Expected value of } Y = \text{E}[Y] = a + bX$$

where a is a constant, known as the "intercept constant" because it is the point on the Y axis where the Y axis is intercepted by the regression line;

b is the slope of the regression line, and is known as the **regression coefficient**;

X is the value of the variable X; and

$\text{E}[Y]$ is the expected value of the variable Y.

Once the values of a and b have been established, the expected value of Y can be predicted for any given value of X. For example, Zito & Reid (1978) showed that the hepatic clearance rate of lidocaine (Y, in ml/min/kg) can be predicted from the hepatic clearance rate of indocyanine green dye (X, in ml/min/kg), according to the equation $Y = 0.30 + 1.07X$, thus enabling anesthesiologists to reduce the risk of lidocaine overdosage by testing clearance of the dye.

Multiple regression

Other techniques generate **multiple regression** equations, in which more than one variable is used to predict the expected value of Y, thus increasing the overall percentage of variance in Y that can be accounted for. For example, Rubin *et al* (1986) found that the birth weight of a baby (Y, in grams) can be partly predicted from the number of cigarettes smoked on a daily basis by both the baby's mother (X_1) and the baby's father (X_2) according to the multiple regression equation $Y = 3385 - 9X_1 - 6X_2$. Other techniques are available to quantify nonlinear relationships among multiple variables. As with correlation, however, it is important to remember that the existence of this kind of statistical association is not in itself evidence of causality.

CHOOSING AN APPROPRIATE INFERENTIAL OR CORRELATIONAL TECHNIQUE

The choice of an appropriate statistical technique for a particular research problem is mainly determined by two factors: the scale of measurement and the type of question being asked. USMLE will require familiarity with only those basic techniques that have been covered here (although there are many others). Their uses will now be summarized.

Concerning *nominal scale data*, only one kind of question has been discussed: do the proportions of observations falling in different categories differ significantly from the proportions that would be expected by chance? The appropriate technique for such questions is the **chi-square test**.

Regarding *ordinal scale data*, only one kind of question has been mentioned: is there an association between ordinal position on one ranking and ordinal position on another ranking? The appropriate technique here is the **Spearman rank-order correlation**.

For *interval* or *ratio scale data*, four general kinds of question have been discussed: questions concerning means (What is the true mean of the population? Is one sample mean significantly different from one or more other sample means?); questions concerning variances (Are the variances in two samples significantly different?); and questions concerning association (To what degree are two variables correlated?).

Three ways of answering questions concerning *means* of interval or ratio scale data have been examined—*t*-tests, *z*-tests, and ANOVA. When the question involves only *one* or *two* means, or making only *one* comparison, a **t-test** will normally be used. Therefore, questions concerning estimation of a population mean, or testing a hypothesis about a population mean, or comparing two sample means with each other, will normally be answered by using *t*. Alternatively, provided that $n \geq 100$, or if the standard deviation of the population is known, a **z-test** may be used with virtually identical results.

When the question involves *more than two* means, or making *more than one* comparison, the appropriate technique is **analysis of variance** (ANOVA), together with **F-tests**, followed by *post hoc* **tests** of various types (if ANOVA has found some significant effects).

One way of answering questions about *variances* has been covered: the **F-test** tests for significant differences between variances.

Two ways of assessing the *degree of association* between two interval or ratio scale variables have been discussed. To evaluate the strength and direction of the relationship, **Pearson product-moment correlation** is used, together with a form of *t*-test to test the null hypothesis that the relationship does not exist in the population. To make predictions about the value of one variable on the basis of the other, **regression** techniques are used.

Table 4-1 summarizes the range of inferential and correlational techniques that have been covered. This table should be memorized to answer typical USMLE questions that require choosing the correct test or technique for a given research situation.

Table 4-1

SCALE OF DATA

		Nominal	Ordinal	Interval or Ratio
Q U E S T I O N S	Differences in proportion	χ^2		
	One or two means			*t*-test (or *z*-test if *n* >100)
C O N C E R N I N G	More than two means			ANOVA with *F*-tests and *post hoc* tests
	Variances			*F*-test
	Association		Spearman ρ	Pearson *r*
	Predicting the value of a variable			Regression

5

Research Methods

Medical researchers typically aim to discover the relationship between one or more events or characteristics (e.g., being exposed to a toxic substance, having a family history of a certain disease, or taking a certain drug) and others (e.g., contracting or recovering from a certain illness). All these events or characteristics are called **variables**.

In any type of research, variables may be either **dependent** or **independent**. Independent variables are presumed to be the *causes* of changes in other variables, which are called the dependent variables because they are presumed to *depend* on the values of the independent variables. Research typically attempts to uncover the relationship between independent variables and dependent variables.

EXPERIMENTAL STUDIES

The relationship between dependent and independent variables can be investigated in two ways: by means of **experimental** studies or **nonexperimental** studies (also called **observational** studies). In experimental work the researcher exercises control over the independent variables, deliberately manipulating them—so experimental studies are sometimes called **intervention** studies. In nonexperimental studies, nature is simply allowed to take its course.

For example, in studying the effectiveness of a particular drug for a certain disease, the administration or nonadministration of the drug is the independent variable, whereas the resulting severity of the disease constitutes the dependent variable, because it is presumed to depend on whether the drug has been used or not.

In an *experimental* investigation of the drug's effectiveness, the investigator would intervene, giving the drug to one group of patients but not to another group. In a *nonexperimental* investigation, the researcher would simply observe different patients who had or had not taken the drug in the normal course of events.

As the example suggests, the hallmark of the experimental method is manipulation or intervention. Properly conducted experiments are the most powerful way of establishing cause-and-effect relationships between independent and dependent variables. But they do have disadvantages: in many cases experiments may be unethical because they may expose subjects to serious physical or mental harm; and they become impractical if the cause–effect relationship is one that takes a long time to appear.

If it is hypothesized that it takes 15 years of heavy alcohol drinking to cause cirrhosis of the liver, it would be unethical and impractical to conduct an experiment by administering heavy doses of alcohol to subjects for this length of time to observe the outcome. However, a researcher could investigate this hypothesis observationally by finding people who have done this in the ordinary course of events.

Clinical trials

The experimental method in medical research commonly takes the form of the **clinical trial**, which attempts to evaluate the effects of a treatment. Clinical trials aim to isolate one factor (such as a new drug) and examine its contribution to patients' health by holding all other factors as constant as possible. Apart from manipulation or intervention, clinical trials typically have two other characteristics: they utilize **control groups** and involve **randomization**. Hence, they are often termed **randomized controlled clinical trials**.

Control groups

Patients in clinical trials are divided into two general groups. One group is the **experimental** group, which is given the treatment under investigation; the other group is the **control** group, which is treated in exactly the same way except that it is not given the treatment. Any difference that appears between the two groups at the end of the study can then be attributed to the treatment under investigation. Control groups, therefore, help to eliminate alternative explanations for a study's results.

> For example, if a drug were found to eliminate all symptoms of an illness in a group of patients in 1 month, it could be argued that the symptoms would have disappeared spontaneously in this period of time even if the drug had not been used. But if a similar group of patients were used as a control group, did not receive the drug, and experienced no improvement in their symptoms, this alternative explanation is untenable.

The two main types of control groups used in medical research are the **no-treatment** control group and the **placebo** control group. A no-treatment control group is the kind used in the previous example: the control group patients receive no treatment at all. This leaves open the possibility that the patients whose symptoms were removed by the drug were responding not to the specific pharmacologic properties of the drug, but to the nonspecific placebo effect that is part of any treatment. By giving an inert placebic treatment to the patients in the control group, this explanation can be eliminated, and the effectiveness of the drug would have to be attributed to its pharmacologic properties.

In studies of this kind, it is obviously important that patients do not know if they are receiving the real drug or the placebo; if patients taking the placebo knew that they were not receiving the real drug, the placebo effect would be greatly reduced or eliminated in this group. It is also important that the physicians or nurses administering the drug and the researchers who assess the patients' outcomes do not know which patients are taking the drug and that are taking the placebo—if they did, this knowledge could cause conscious or unconscious bias which might affect their interactions with and evaluations of the patients. The patients and all those involved with them in the conduct of the experiment should therefore be "blind" as to which patients are in which group. These kinds of studies are therefore called **double-blind** studies.

It is not always possible to perform a double-blind study. For example, in an experiment comparing the effectiveness of a drug versus a surgical procedure, it would be hard if not impossible to keep the patient "blind" as to which treatment he or she received; but it would be possible for the outcome to be measured by a "blind" rater, who might perform laboratory tests or interviews with the patient without knowing to which group the patient belonged. Such a study would be called a **single-blind** study.

Under some circumstances truly controlled experiments may not be possible. In research on the effectiveness of psychotherapy, for example, patients who are placed in a no-treatment control group may well receive help from friends, family, clergy, self-help books, and so on, and would therefore not constitute a true no-treatment control. In this case, the study would be called a **partially controlled** clinical trial.

Controlled experiments pose ethical problems if there is good reason to believe that the treatment under investigation is either a beneficial or a harmful one. In the 1950s, experiments on the effects of oxygen on premature babies were opposed on the grounds that the control group babies would be deprived of a beneficial treatment; later, when it became strongly suspected that excessive oxygen was a cause of retrolental fibroplasia, similar experiments were opposed because the *experimental* group might be subjected to a harmful treatment. Under some circumstances it may be unethical to continue a controlled experiment once it has begun to show that the treatment is indeed effective. In 1986, for example, a controlled trial of the AIDS drug zidovudine (AZT, Retrovir®) was halted: it was believed that it was unethical to deprive the control group patients of an apparently effective drug (Barnes, 1986). The argument that it is unethical to deprive patients of *any* treatment that has the potential to save them from an otherwise certain death carries obvious moral weight; however, this may preclude the conduct of well-controlled experiments that effectively test new drugs.

Randomization

Randomization means that patients are randomly assigned to different groups (i.e., to the experimental and control groups) to equalize the effects of extraneous variables.

In a controlled trial of a new drug, it would be absurd to assign all the male patients or all the less severely diseased patients to the drug group, and all the females or all the more severely diseased patients to the control group. If this were done, any difference in outcome between the two groups could be attributed to differences between the sexes or pretreatment severities of the disease in the two groups rather than to the drug itself. In this kind of situation, patient gender and disease severity are called **confounding variables**, because they contribute differently and inextricably to the two groups. To avoid confounding effects, patients are normally assigned randomly to the two groups, so that the different independent variables (in this case, gender, disease severity, and receiving the drug) are not systematically related.

Allocating patients randomly to the different experimental groups guards against bias; true randomization means that the groups should be similar with respect to gender, disease severity, age, occupation, and any other variable that may differentially affect response to the experimental intervention.

However, randomization cannot *guarantee* that the groups are similar in all important ways. An alternative method of ensuring that the experimental and control groups are similar is to use **matching**, in which each patient in the experimental group is paired with a patient in the control group who matches the experimental patient closely on all relevant characteristics. If gender, race, and age were important factors influencing the course of the disease being studied, each experimental patient would be matched with a control patient of the same gender, race, and age—thus, any resulting differences between the two groups could not be attributed to differences in gender, race, or age.

Sometimes a combination of randomization and matching techniques is used. The population under study is first divided, or **stratified**, into subgroups that are internally homogeneous with respect to the important factors (e.g., race, age, disease severity). Then, equal numbers of patients within each subgroup are randomly allocated to the experimental and control groups. The two groups are therefore similar, but their exact membership is still a result of randomization. This technique is therefore called **stratified randomization**.

In the previously described methods, comparisons are being made between patients (or subjects) in one group and patients in the other group; these studies are therefore called **between-subjects** designs. An alternative approach is to use each patient as his or her *own* control, which means that comparisons are being made *within* each subject, a **within-subjects** design, and the control group is a **same-subject** control group. This method solves the problem of achieving comparability between the control and experimental groups.

A common type of research using the within-subjects approach is the **crossover** design. Here half the patients receive the placebo for a period of time, followed by the experimental treatment; the other half receive the treatment first, then the placebo. This is also called a **Latin square** design. If there is a danger of a "carryover" effect (for example, if the treatment is a drug that may continue to have some effect after it is withdrawn), then there can be a **washout** period in between the drug and placebo phases, during which no treatment is given.

Figure 5-1 illustrates a crossover design with washout. One group of patients receives the drug for 1 month, and then "crosses over" to receive the placebo after 1 month's washout. The other group follows this pattern in reverse order. The efficacy of the drug is determined by comparing the effects of the drug and placebo *within each patient*. This kind of design is also called a **repeated measures** design, because the measurements (of the dependent variable, such as the severity of the patients' symptoms) are repeated within each patient at different times, and results are analyzed by comparing the measurements that have been repeated on each patient.

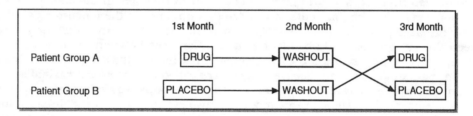

Figure 5-1

NONEXPERIMENTAL STUDIES

Nonexperimental (or observational) studies fall into two general classes: **descriptive studies** and **analytic studies**.

Descriptive studies aim to describe the occurrence and distribution of diseases or other phenomena. They do not try to offer explanations or test a theory or a hypothesis; they merely generate a description of the frequency of the disease or other phenomenon of interest according to the places, times, and people involved. As a result, they are often the first method used to study a particular disease—hence, they are also called **exploratory studies**—and they may serve to generate hypotheses for analytic studies to test. Well-known examples of modern descriptive studies include those of Legionnaire's disease following its first recognized outbreak in 1976, and early studies of AIDS showing that male homosexuals, intravenous drug abusers, and hemophiliacs were at risk. In both these cases the true nature of the disease was unknown at the time, but the findings of descriptive studies generated useful hypotheses.

Analytic studies aim to test hypotheses or to provide explanations about a disease or other phenomenon—hypotheses or explanations that are often drawn from earlier descriptive studies.

Descriptive and analytic studies are not always entirely distinguishable in practice; for example, a large-scale descriptive study may provide such clear data that it may itself provide an answer to questions or give clear support to a particular hypothesis.

Both kinds of nonexperimental studies, whether descriptive or analytic, employ one of four principal research designs: they may be **cohort studies**, **case-control studies**, **case series studies**, or **prevalence surveys**.

Cohort studies

Cohort studies focus on factors related to the development of a disease. In these studies, a **cohort** (a group of people) who do *not* have the disease of interest is selected and then observed for an extended period of time. Some members of the cohort will already have been exposed to a suspected risk factor for the disease, and others will eventually become exposed; by following them all, the relationship between the risk factors and the eventual outcomes can be seen. This kind of study therefore allows the incidence and natural history of a disease to be studied.

Cohort studies may be loosely termed **follow-up** or **longitudinal** studies because they follow people over a prolonged period of time, tracing any changes through repeated observation. They are also called **prospective** studies because people are followed forward from a particular point in time, so the researcher is "prospecting" or looking for new data about events that are yet to happen. In addition, cohort studies are sometimes called **incidence** studies because they look for the incidence of new cases of the disease over time.

> A famous example of a cohort study is the Framingham Study, which was begun in 1949. This started with a cohort of over 5000 people in Framingham, Massachusetts, who were free of coronary heart disease (CHD). The individuals in the cohort were reexamined every 2 years for a period of over 30 years. This study succeeded in identifying the major physical risk factors for CHD.

> Another example is the Western Collaborative Group Study (WCGS), which followed a cohort of over 5000 heart disease–free California males for 7 years, showing that type A personality was strongly associated with increased risk of CHD. (This study has subsequently been extended to a 21-year follow-up, with somewhat contradictory results.)

Cohort studies have a number of significant advantages:

1. When a true experiment cannot be conducted (whether for ethical or practical reasons), cohort studies are the best form of investigation; their findings are often extremely valuable.

2. They are the only method by which the absolute risk of contracting a disease can be established, and they can help to answer one of the most clinically relevant questions: if someone is exposed to a certain suspected risk factor, is that person more likely to contract the disease? Cohort studies may also reveal the existence of protective factors such as regular exercise and diet.

3. Because cohort studies are prospective, the assessment of risk factors in these studies is unbiased by the outcome. If the Framingham Study were retrospective, for example, people's recollection of their diet and smoking habits could have been biased by the fact that they already have CHD (this effect is known as **recall bias**). In addition, the chronologic relationship between the risk factors and the disease is clear; if the WCGS were retrospective, it might be unclear whether people developed a type A personality style *after* contracting CHD, rather than beforehand.

4. For those individuals in a cohort who ultimately contract the disease of interest, data concerning their exposure to suspected risk factors have already been collected. But in a retrospective study this may not be possible—again, if the Framingham Study were retrospective, it might have been impossible to obtain accurate information about the diet and smoking habits of people who had already died. And if the WCGS were retrospective, it would have been difficult if not impossible to assess the personality of people who had already died. Other types of studies are often unable to include people who die of the disease in question—often the most important people to study.

5. Information about suspected risk factors collected in cohort studies can be used to examine the relationship between these risk factors and *many* diseases; therefore, a study designed as an analytic investigation of one disease may simultaneously serve as a valuable descriptive study of several other diseases.

Cohort studies have some important disadvantages:

1. They are time consuming, laborious, and expensive to conduct; members of the cohort must be followed for a long time (often for many years) before a sufficient number of them get the disease of interest. It will often be very expensive and difficult to keep track of a large number of people for several years, and it may be many years before results are produced, especially in the case of diseases that take a long time to appear after exposure to a risk factor.

2. They are usually impractical for rare diseases. For example, if one case of a disease occurs in every 10,000 people, then 100,000 people will have to be followed for 10 cases to eventually appear. However, if a particular cohort with a high rate of the disease can be identified, such as an occupational cohort (a group of people engaged in the same type of work), then a disease that is rare in the general population can still be studied by the cohort method. Classic examples of this include studies of scrotal cancer among chimney sweeps and of bladder cancer among dye workers.

Case-control studies

Whereas cohort studies examine people who are all initially free of the disease of interest, **case-control** studies compare people who *do* have the disease (the cases) with otherwise similar people who do *not* have the disease (the controls).

Case-control studies therefore start with the outcome, or dependent variable (the presence or absence of the disease), and then look back into the past for possible independent variables that may have caused the disease to see if a possible or suspected cause or risk factor was present more frequently in people with the disease than in those without. Hence, they are also called **retrospective** studies.

One classic exploratory case-control study uncovered the relationship between maternal exposure to diethylstilbestrol (DES) and clear-cell adenocarcinoma of the vagina in young women (Herbst *et al*, 1971). Eight patients with this rare cancer were each compared with four matched cancer-free controls. Looking back at their individual and maternal histories, no significant differences appeared between the cases and the controls on a wide range of variables, but it was found that mothers of seven of the eight cases had taken DES in early pregnancy, 15 to 20 years ago, whereas none of the 32 controls' mothers had done so.

Case-control studies offer some significant advantages:

1. They can be performed relatively quickly and cheaply (especially in comparison with cohort studies), even for rare diseases or diseases that take a long time to appear (as the previous example shows). Because of this, cohort studies are the most important way of investigating rare diseases and are typically used in the early exploration of a disease.

2. They require comparatively few subjects.

3. They allow multiple potential causes of a disease to be investigated.

Case-control studies also have a number of disadvantages and are particularly subject to bias:

1. People's recall of their past behaviors or risk-factor exposure may be biased by the fact that they now have the disease.

2. The only cases that can be investigated are those of people who have been identified and diagnosed—undiagnosed or asymptomatic cases would be missed by this kind of study. People who have already died of the disease of interest cannot be questioned about their past behaviors and exposure to risk factors.

3. Selection of a comparable control group is a difficult task that relies entirely on the researcher's judgment.

4. Case-control studies cannot determine the rates or the risk of the disease in exposed and nonexposed people.

Case series studies

A **case series** simply describes the clinical presentation of a disease in a number of patients at a particular time. It does not follow the patients for a period of time, and it uses no control or comparison group.

A case series therefore cannot establish a cause–effect relationship, and the fact that there is no control group with which to compare the cases means that the validity of its findings is entirely a matter for the reader to decide. For example, a report that 8 of 10 patients with a certain disease have a history of exposure to some particular risk factor may be extremely useful or almost worthless, depending on the circumstances and the reader's own judgment.

Despite these serious shortcomings, case series studies are commonly used to present new information about patients with a rare disease, and they may stimulate new hypotheses and research about a particular disease or phenomenon. They can be carried out by almost any physician who carefully observes and records patient information. A **case report** is a special form of case series in which only one patient is described—it too may be very valuable or virtually worthless.

Prevalence surveys

A **prevalence survey** is a survey of a whole population, including diseased and disease-free individuals. It aims to determine the proportion of people who are diseased (this is the **prevalence** of the disease; see Figure 6-1) and to examine the relationship between the disease and other characteristics of the population. Because prevalence surveys are based on a single examination of the population at a particular point in time and do not follow the population over time, they are also called **cross-sectional** studies, in distinction to longitudinal cohort studies.

Prevalence surveys are common in the medical literature. Examples include a study of the prevalence of CHD in a community—the results of this study could be compared with the results of a similar study in a different community with different dietary or exercise habits; or a study examining the prevalence of respiratory disease in a city—which could then be compared with a survey in another city with lower levels of cigarette consumption or air pollution.

Prevalence surveys suffer from a number of disadvantages. Because they look at existing cases of a disease, and not at the occurrence of new cases, they are likely to over-represent diseases of long duration and to under-represent short-lived diseases. They may be unusable for acute diseases, which few if any people suffered from at the moment they were questioned or examined. In addition, people suffering from some types of disease may leave the community under study, or may be institutionalized, causing them to be excluded from the survey. Findings of prevalence surveys must be interpreted cautiously; the mere fact that two variables (such as increased exercise and reduced illness) are found to be associated does not mean that they are causally related.

Although they may be expensive and laborious to carry out, prevalence surveys are common because they have the potential to produce very valuable data about a wide range of diseases, behaviors, and characteristics, which can be used to generate several hypotheses for more analytic studies to examine.

6

Statistics in Epidemiology

Epidemiology is the study of the distribution, determinants, and dynamics of health and disease in populations or groups of people in relation to their environment and ways of living. These phenomena can be statistically described by means of **rates**, which will be discussed in the first part of this chapter, and by **measures of risk**, which will be described in the second part.

RATES

All rates consist of a numerator (usually the number of people with a particular condition) and a denominator (usually the number of people at risk), and they usually specify or imply a unit of time. The most important rates are **incidence** and **prevalence** (which are both measures of **morbidity**), **mortality**, and **case-fatality**.

Incidence

The **incidence** of a disease is the number of new cases occurring in a particular time period. The incidence rate is therefore the ratio of new cases of the disease to the total number of people at risk:

$$\text{Incidence rate} = \frac{\text{number of new cases of the disease}}{\text{total number of people at risk}} \text{ per unit of time}$$

The incidence rate is often stated per 100,000 of the population at risk, or as a percentage; the unit of time may be 1 day, 1 week, 1 year, or any other suitable time period. Incidence rates are found by the use of cohort studies, which are therefore sometimes also known as incidence studies (see Chapter 5).

Prevalence

The **prevalence** of a disease is the number of people affected by it at a particular moment in time. The prevalence rate is therefore the ratio of the number of people with the disease to the total number of people at risk:

$$\text{Prevalence rate} = \frac{\text{number of people with the disease}}{\text{total number of people at risk}} \text{ at a particular time}$$

Like incidence rates, prevalence rates are often stated per 100,000 people, or as a percentage. They are generally found by prevalence surveys.

Prevalence is an appropriate measure of the burden of a relatively stable chronic condition (such as hypertension or diabetes) on the population. However, it is not generally appropriate for acute illnesses, as it depends on the average duration of the disease. Prevalence is equal to the *incidence multiplied by the average duration of the disease*, so an increased prevalence rate may merely reflect increased duration of an acute illness, rather than suggesting that members of the population are at greater risk of contracting the disease.

Incidence and prevalence are both measures of **morbidity**, or the rate of illness.

Mortality

Mortality is the number of deaths. The mortality rate is the ratio of the number of people dying (whether of a specific disease or of all causes) to the total number of people at risk:

$$\text{Mortality rate} = \frac{\text{total number of deaths}}{\text{total number of people at risk}} \text{ per unit of time}$$

Like incidence and prevalence, mortality rates may be expressed as a percentage, or the number of deaths per 1000 or 100,000 people. The unit of time may be any convenient period. Mortality is actually a special form of incidence in which the event in question is death rather than contraction of a disease. Mortality figures are likely to be more accurate than incidence figures, because deaths are always recorded whereas episodes of illness are not. However, accurate records of causes of death are often unavailable, and mortality rates will not reflect the total burden of illness except in the case of diseases that are always fatal.

The "epidemiologist's bathtub"

The relationships between incidence, prevalence, and mortality in any disease can be visualized with the aid of the "epidemiologist's bathtub," shown in Figure 6-1. The flow of water through the faucet into the bathtub is analogous to incidence, representing the arrival of new cases of the disease; the level of water in the tub represents the prevalence, or number of cases of the disease existing at any given point in time; the flow of water out through the plughole represents mortality; and the evaporation of water represents either cure or a natural progression to recovery.

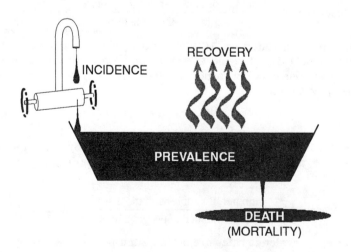

Figure 6-1

Alzheimer's disease provides an example of the application of the "bathtub." There is a roughly constant incidence of Alzheimer's disease (inflow of water), and modern medicine is able to keep people with the disorder alive for longer, thus reducing the mortality rate from the disease (partially blocking the plughole); however, because there is no cure for the disease, and it never progresses to recovery, the result is clearly an increased prevalence (increased water level)—which is apparent in the United States today.

Case fatality

The **case fatality rate** (CFR) is the ratio of the number of people dying in a particular episode of a disease to the total number of episodes of the disease, expressed as a percentage:

$$CFR = \frac{\text{total number of people dying in an episode of the disease}}{\text{total number of episodes of the disease}} \times 100$$

The CFR is a measure of the prognosis, in terms of life or death, for an episode of a given disease, because it shows the likelihood of one episode or occurrence of it resulting in death.

Adjustment of rates

Researchers may want to compare rates across different populations, e.g., to compare the incidence of a disease in one city or country with that in another. However, if the populations differ significantly on one or more factors that are relevant to the illness in question, the comparison will be a biased one.

> A researcher wants to compare the prevalence of AIDS in two cities of equal size. City A has a large proportion of young people (under the age of 45) whereas city B does not— so it would not be surprising if city A had a higher prevalence of AIDS than city B. However, due to the confounding effects of the different age structures of the two cities' populations, this prevalence rate alone tells the researcher nothing about any real *underlying* difference in the prevalence of AIDS in the two cities.

The biasing influence of a confounding variable (such as age) can be removed by the technique of **adjustment** (or **standardization**) **of rates**. This involves calculating rates for the two populations as if they were both the same in terms of the factors (such as age) that are relevant to the disease, so that their rates of the disease can be compared:

> Assume that the prevalence of AIDS in city A is 38 per 100,000, whereas in city B it is 29 per 100,000. Because city A has a much larger proportion of young people (80%) than city B (40%), the difference in their rates of AIDS may be merely due to their differing age structures.

> To examine this possibility, the researcher needs to know the *age-specific* prevalence rates of the disease in the two cities. They are as shown (per 100,000) in Table 6-1.

Table 6-1

	City A	City B
Under age 45	40	50
Over age 45	30	15

It is now possible to *age-adjust* the rates to equalize the weight given to age in the two cities. This is done by applying the known rates in each age-group to either a real or a hypothetical standard population that has either a known or an arbitrary age structure. This standard population could be almost any population; it is common to use the age distribution of the United States as a whole or the total population of the two communities being studied. In this example, the latter will be done. Because the two cities are of equal size, and 80% of the population of one is young whereas only 40% of the population of the other is young, then 60% of their *total* population is young and 40% of it is old.

The overall age-adjusted prevalence of AIDS in city A is found by multiplying the known prevalence of AIDS in this city's young group (40 per 100,000) by 0.6 (because 60% of the total standard population are young), and adding this to the product of the known prevalence of AIDS in the city's old population (30 per 100,000) times 0.4 (40% of the total standard population are old):

$$(40 \times 0.6) + (30 \times 0.4) = 24 + 12 = 36 \text{ per } 100,000$$

The same is then done for city B. City B's prevalence of 50 per 100,000 among the young is multiplied by 0.6, and this is added to the prevalence figure among the old (15 per 100,000) times 0.4, giving the total age-adjusted prevalence in city B:

$$(50 \times 0.6) + (15 \times 0.4) = 30 + 6 = 36 \text{ per } 100,000$$

The age-adjusted prevalence of AIDS in the two cities is therefore identical, demonstrating that the apparent difference in the prevalence of AIDS is attributable merely to the difference in their age structures.

This kind of process of adjustment (or standardization) can be done not only for age, but also for any other relevant factor that differs substantially between two populations that are being compared. Adjustment can be made for two or more factors simultaneously—for example, if city A had many more IV drug abusers than city B, this difference could also be adjusted for.

MEASUREMENT OF RISK

Information about the risk of contracting a given disease is of great value in medicine. The knowledge that something is a risk factor for a disease can be used in several ways: to help prevent the disease; to help predict its future incidence and prevalence; to help diagnose the disease (diagnostic suspicions will be aroused if it is known that a patient was exposed to the risk factor); and to help establish the cause of a disease of unknown etiology.

Absolute risk

The fundamental measure of risk is incidence. The incidence of a disease is, in fact, the **absolute risk** of contracting it. For example, if the incidence of a disease is 10 per 1000 people per annum, then the absolute risk of a person actually contracting it is also 10 per 1000 per annum, or 1% per annum.

However, it is useful to go beyond absolute risk and to compare the incidence of a disease in different groups of people to find out if exposure to a suspected risk factor (such as cigarettes) increases the risk of contracting a certain disease (such as lung cancer). A number of different comparisons of risk can be made, including **relative risk**, **attributable risk**, and the **odds ratio**. All these are called **measures of effect**—they aim to measure the effect of being exposed to a risk factor on the risk of contracting a disease.

Theoretically, the ideal way of determining the effect of a risk factor is by means of a controlled experiment, but this is hardly ever ethical. The best alternative approach is the cohort (prospective) study, in which the incidence of disease in exposed and nonexposed people can be directly observed.

One of the main goals of such research (such as the Framingham Study and the Western Group Collaborative Study, described briefly in Chapter 5) is to find the extent to which the risk of contracting the disease in question is increased by exposure to the risk factor. The two measures that show this are **relative risk** and **attributable risk**.

Relative risk

Relative risk states by how many times exposure to the risk factor increases the risk of contracting the disease. It is therefore the ratio of the incidence of the disease among exposed persons to the incidence of the disease among unexposed persons:

$$\text{Relative risk} = \frac{\text{incidence of the disease among persons exposed to the risk factor}}{\text{incidence of the disease among persons not exposed to the risk factor}}$$

As an example, Table 6-2 reports the results of a hypothetical cohort study in which 1008 heavy smokers and 1074 nonsmokers were followed for a number of years to observe the incidence of lung cancer among them. It can be seen that the incidence of lung cancer over the total time period of the study among people exposed to the risk factor (heavy cigarette smoking) is 283/1008, or .28 (28%), whereas the incidence among those not exposed is 64/1074, or .06 (6%). The relative risk is therefore .28/.06, or 4.67, showing that people who smoked cigarettes heavily were 4.67 times more likely to contract lung cancer than were nonsmokers during the period of the study. (Note that this not a measure of *absolute* risk—it states nothing about the likelihood of heavy smokers contracting cancer in absolute terms.)

Table 6-2

RISK	DISEASE OUTCOME		
	Lung Cancer	No Lung Cancer	Total
Exposed (heavy smokers)	283	725	1008
Nonexposed (nonsmokers)	64	1010	1074
Total	347	1735	2082

Because relative risk is a ratio of risks, it is sometimes called the **risk ratio**, or **morbidity ratio**. In the case of outcomes involving death, rather than just disease, it may also be called the **mortality ratio**.

Attributable risk

The attributable risk is the *additional* incidence of a disease that is attributable to the risk factor in question. It is equal to the incidence of the disease in the exposed persons minus the incidence of the disease in the nonexposed persons. In the previous example, the attributable risk is equal to .28 – .06, or .22 (22%)—in other words, 22% of the 28% incidence of lung cancer among the heavy smokers in this study is attributable to smoking. The other 6% is the "background" incidence of the disease—its incidence among those not exposed to this particular risk factor. Attributable risk is sometimes called **risk difference**, because it is the difference in the risks or incidences of the disease between the two groups of people.

Odds ratio

Relative risk and attributable risk both require the use of cohort (prospective) studies, as shown previously. However, as noted in Chapter 5, cohort studies are generally expensive, time-consuming, and laborious to conduct, and are therefore often impractical.

A common alternative is to use a case-control (retrospective) study, which compares people *with* the disease (cases) with otherwise similar people *without* the disease (controls), attempting to look back into the past to see if a possible risk factor is found more frequently among the cases than the controls (see Chapter 5). If the proportion of people exposed to the possible risk factor is greater among the cases, then the risk factor is implicated as a cause of the disease. The **odds ratio** (or **relative odds**) is a measure of these relative proportions—it is the ratio of the odds that a case was exposed to the risk factor *to* the odds that a control was exposed to the risk factor:

$$\text{Odds ratio} = \frac{\text{odds that a case was exposed to the risk factor}}{\text{odds that a control was exposed to the risk factor}}$$

Because the proportion of people in the study who do have the disease is determined by the researcher's choice, and not by the actual proportion in the population, case-control studies cannot determine the incidence or prevalence of a disease; thus, they cannot determine the risk of contracting a disease. The odds ratio must therefore be used instead of relative risk when analyzing case-control data instead of cohort data.

For example, the hypothetical data that were used to illustrate the calculation of relative risk in Table 6-2 can be used, but now assume that these data were generated by a case-control study in which history of prior exposure to the risk factor (cigarette smoking) was compared between 347 cases (with lung cancer) and 1735 controls (without lung cancer).

Table 6-3

	DISEASE OUTCOME		
RISK	Lung Cancer (cases)	No Lung Cancer (controls)	Total
Exposed (heavy smokers)	283 (A)	725 (B)	1008
Nonexposed (nonsmokers)	64 (C)	1010 (D)	1074
Total	347	1735	2082

As defined previously, the odds ratio is the ratio of the odds that a case was exposed *to* the odds that a control was exposed; it can be shown[1] that this is equal to

$$\frac{\text{number of cases exposed to risk factor }(A) \times \text{number of controls not exposed }(D)}{\text{number of controls exposed to risk factor }(B) \times \text{number of cases not exposed }(C)}$$

Table 6-3 shows that:

283 of the cases were exposed to the risk factor *(A)*

725 of the controls were exposed to the risk factor *(B)*

64 of the cases were not exposed to the risk factor *(C)*

1010 of the controls were not exposed to the risk factor *(D)*

The odds ratio is, therefore, $\dfrac{283 \times 1010}{725 \times 64} = \dfrac{285830}{46400} = 6.16$

In other words, among the people studied, a person with lung cancer was 6.16 times more likely to have been exposed to the risk factor (cigarette smoking) than was a person without lung cancer.

Note that an odds ratio of 1 indicates that a person with the disease is no more likely to have been exposed to the risk factor than is a person without the disease, suggesting that the risk factor is not related to the disease. An odds ratio of less than 1 indicates that a person with the disease is *less* likely to have been exposed to the risk factor than is a person without the disease, implying that the risk factor is actually a *protective* factor against the disease.

In some ways the odds ratio is similar to the relative risk: both figures demonstrate the strength of the association between the risk factor and the disease, albeit in different ways. As a result of their similarities, the odds ratio is sometimes called **estimated relative risk**— it provides a reasonably good estimate of relative risk *provided* that the incidence of the disease is low (which is usually true of chronic diseases), and that the cases and controls examined in the study are representative of people with and without the disease in the population.

NOTE

[1] The derivation of this is as follows. Referring to the cells in Table 6-3, the odds that a case was exposed are $\dfrac{A/(A+C)}{C/(A+C)} = A/C$.

The odds that a control was exposed are $\dfrac{B/(B+D)}{D/(B+D)} = B/D$.

The ratio of these odds is $\dfrac{A/C}{B/D}$,

which, when cross-multiplied, becomes $\dfrac{A \times D}{B \times C}$.

7

Statistics in
Medical Decision Making

Medical decision making frequently involves using tests or quantitative data of various kinds. Any physician using a diagnostic test—whether it is a physical test, a laboratory test of some aspect of a patient's functioning, or a screening test being used on a whole population—will want to know how good the test is.

This is a complex question, as the qualities and characteristics of tests can be evaluated in a variety of different important ways. To assess the quality of a diagnostic test, it is necessary as a minimum to know its **validity** and **reliability**, its **sensitivity** and **specificity**, and its **positive** and **negative predictive values**. Similarly, when using quantitative test results—such as measurements of fasting blood sugar, serum cholesterol, blood urea nitrogen, and so on—the physician will need to know the **accuracy** and **precision** of the measurement as well as the normal **reference values** for the variable in question. This chapter discusses each of these concepts in turn.

VALIDITY

The validity of a test is the extent to which it actually tests what it claims to test—in other words, how closely its results correspond to the real state of affairs. The validity of a diagnostic or screening test is, therefore, its ability to show which individuals have the disease in question and which do not. To be truly valid, a test should be highly sensitive, specific (see page 71), and unbiased. Quantitatively, the validity of a diagnostic or screening test is the proportion of all test results that are correct, as determined by comparison with an accepted standard (sometimes called the **gold standard**) which is known to be totally correct.

Validity is synonymous with accuracy. As stated in Chapter 2, the accuracy of a figure or measurement is the degree to which it is immune from systematic error or bias. To the extent that a measurement or test result is free from systematic error or bias, it is accurate and valid.

RELIABILITY

Reliability is synonymous with repeatability and reproducibility—it is the level of agreement between repeated measurements of the same variable. Hence, it is also called **test–retest reliability**. In the case of a test of a stable variable, it can be quantified in terms of the correlation between measurements made at different times. This is the test's "reliability coefficient."

Reliability corresponds to precision, defined in Chapter 2 as the degree to which a figure is immune from random variation. A test that is affected very little by random variation will obviously produce very similar results when it is used to measure a stable variable at different times. A reliable test is therefore a consistent, stable, and dependable one.

The reliability or repeatability of a test influences the extent to which a single measurement may be taken as a definitive guide for making a diagnosis. In the case of a highly reliable test, one measurement alone may be sufficient to allow a physician to diagnose with confidence; however, if the test is unreliable in any way, this may not be possible. The inherent instability of many biomedical variables (such as blood pressure) often makes it necessary to repeat a measurement at different times and to use the mean of these results to obtain a reliable measurement and make a confident diagnosis.

In practice, neither validity nor reliability is usually in question in routine hospital laboratory testing. Standard laboratory tests have been carefully validated by their originators and manufacturers, and careful quality control procedures and instrumentation (including the increasing use of automated testing systems) in the laboratory ensures reliability.

A test or measurement may be reliable or precise without necessarily being valid or accurate. For example, it would be possible to measure the circumference of a person's skull with great reliability and precision, but this would certainly not constitute a valid assessment of the person's intelligence.

Bias may also cause a reliable and precise measurement to be invalid. A laboratory balance, for example, may weigh very precisely, with very little variation between repeated weighings of the same object; but if it has not been zeroed properly, all its measurements may be 3 mg high, causing all its results to be biased, and hence inaccurate and invalid.

Conversely, a measurement may be valid, yet unreliable. In medicine this is often due to the inherent instability of the variable being measured. Repeated measurements of a patient's blood pressure may vary considerably; yet if all these measurements cluster around one figure, the findings as a whole may accurately represent the true state of affairs (e.g., that a patient is hypertensive).

REFERENCE VALUES

No matter how high the quality of a set of measurements, they do not in themselves permit the physician to make a diagnosis, even if they are both valid and reliable.

To make a diagnosis, the physician must have some idea of the range of values of the measured variable among normal, healthy people. This range is called the **normal range** or **reference range**, and the limits of this range are the **reference values** with which the physician will compare the values obtained from the patient. (The range between the reference values is sometimes called the **reference interval**.)

How can a valid set of reference values be established? The "normal range" or "reference range" of a biomedical variable is often arbitrarily defined as the middle 95% of the normal (or Gaussian) distribution—in other words, the population mean plus or minus two standard deviations (explained in Chapter 2). The limits of this range, derived from a healthy population, are often taken to be the "reference values." The assumptions being made here are:

1. The 95% of the population that lie within this range are "normal," whereas the 5% beyond it are "abnormal" or "pathologic."

2. The "normal range" for a particular biomedical variable (e.g., serum cholesterol) can be obtained by measuring it in a large representative population of normal,

healthy individuals, thus obtaining a normal distribution; the central 95% of this normal distribution would then be the "normal range."

Although manufacturers of commercial tests may attempt to establish a reference range by testing thousands, or even tens of thousands, of individuals, the practical facts are:

1. There is nothing inherently pathologic about the 5% of the population outside this "normal range"; typically, there are some healthy people who have "abnormally" high or low values. Indeed, in some cases an abnormal value—such as a low serum cholesterol value or a high IQ—may be a positive sign rather than a negative one.

2. Many biologic variables turn out to be skewed rather than normally distributed in the population.

3. The population that is tested to establish the normal range is not usually unambiguously free of disease, because it is difficult to find a large sample of "normal" people who are healthy in every way.

4. If this strictly statistical definition of normality and abnormality were adhered to, all diseases would have the same prevalence rate of 5%.

In practice the normal range and the corresponding reference values presented in a given laboratory's manual often represent a compromise between the statistically derived values and clinical judgment, and may be altered from time to time as the laboratory gains experience with a given test. The values must always be interpreted in the light of other factors that may influence the data obtained about a given patient, such as the patient's age, weight, gender, diet, physical position, and the time of day when the specimen was drawn or the measurement made.

Table 7-1

		DISEASE	
		Present	Absent
TEST RESULT	Positive	True positive (*TP*)	False positive (type II error) (*FP*)
	Negative	False negative (type I error) (*FN*)	True negative (*TN*)

SENSITIVITY AND SPECIFICITY

Sensitivity and specificity are both measures of a test's validity—its ability to correctly detect people with and people without the disease in question. These two concepts are best understood by referring to Table 7-1, which shows the four logical possibilities in diagnostic testing:

TP : A positive test result may be obtained in the case of a person who has the disease; this is a "true positive" finding.

FP : A positive test result may be obtained in the case of a person who does not have the disease; this finding is therefore a "false positive" one, which is a type II error.

FN :   A negative test result may be obtained in the case of a person who does have the disease; this is a "false negative" result, which constitutes a type I error.

TN :   A negative test result may be obtained in the case of a person who does not have the disease; this is a "true negative" result.

Sensitivity

The sensitivity of a test is its ability to detect people who *do* have the disease; it is the percentage of the diseased people who are correctly detected or classified:

$$\text{Sensitivity} = \frac{\text{number testing positive who have the disease } (TP)}{\text{total number tested who have the disease } (TP + FN)} \times 100$$

So a test that is always positive for diseased individuals, identifying *every* diseased person, has a sensitivity of 100%. Therefore, a test that is insensitive leads to missed diagnoses (false negative results), whereas a sensitive test produces few false negative results.

A sensitive test is obviously required in situations in which the consequences of a false negative result is serious, as in the case of a serious condition that is treatable or transmissible. High sensitivity is required of tests used to screen donated blood for HIV, or in the case of cytological screening tests for cervical cancer.

Very sensitive tests are therefore used for *screening* or *ruling out* disease; if the result of a highly sensitive test is negative, it allows the disease to be ruled out with confidence.

Specificity

The specificity of a test is its ability to detect people who *do not* have the disease. It is the percentage of the disease-free people who are correctly classified or detected:

$$\text{Specificity} = \frac{\text{number testing negative who do not have the disease } (TN)}{\text{total number tested who do not have the disease } (FP + TN)} \times 100$$

So a test that is always negative for healthy individuals, identifying *every* nondiseased person, has a specificity of 100%. A test that is low in specificity therefore leads to many false positive diagnoses, whereas a test that is highly specific produces few false positive results.

High specificity is required in situations in which the consequences of a false positive diagnosis are serious: where the diagnosis may lead to the initiation of dangerous, painful, or expensive treatments (as in the case of cancer chemotherapy); where a diagnosis may be unduly alarming (HIV positivity); where a diagnosis may cause a person to make irreversible decisions about his or her living arrangements (Alzheimer's disease); or where a diagnosis may result in a person being stigmatized with an incorrect label (schizophrenia, HIV positivity).

Very specific tests are therefore appropriate for *confirming* or *ruling in* the existence of a disease. If the result of a highly specific test is positive, the disease is almost certainly present.

In clinical practice, sensitivity and specificity are inversely related: an increase in one causes a reduction in the other. This is because the diseased and non-diseased groups of patients lie on a continuum, overlapping each other, rather than forming two totally discrete groups. The tester therefore has to select a "cutoff point" to make a diagnostic decision.

For example, the fasting blood sugar levels of the populations of persons who have diabetes and persons who do not have diabetes might form two overlapping distributions resembling those shown in Figure 7-1.

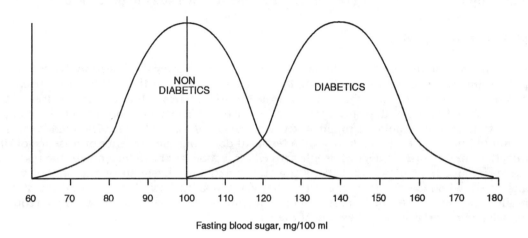

Fasting blood sugar, mg/100 ml

Figure 7-1

It is apparent that when a test of fasting blood sugar is used to diagnose diabetes, the choice of cutoff point will determine the test's sensitivity and specificity.

If the cutoff point were set at 100 mg/100 ml, the test would be 100% sensitive, correctly identifying *every* person with diabetes; but it would have a very low specificity, producing a large number of false positive results—many persons who do not have diabetes would be incorrectly diagnosed as having diabetes. As this suggests, highly sensitive tests are likely to have low specificity. Although they correctly classify the vast majority of diseased people (making few false negative or type I errors), they tend to classify many healthy people incorrectly (making a large number of false positive or type II errors).

If the cutoff point were increased (i.e., moved to the right along the X axis), it is clear that the test's sensitivity would gradually decrease and its specificity would increase until the cutoff point reached 140 mg/100 ml, at which point the test would be 100% specific. At this level it would correctly identify all persons who do not have diabetes, but it would be highly insensitive, incorrectly diagnosing many persons with diabetes as not having diabetes. Highly specific tests are therefore likely to be associated with a high number of false negative (type I) errors.

It is clear from Figure 7-1 that a test can only be 100% sensitive *and* 100% specific if there is no overlap at all between the normal and diseased populations. For example, if no person with diabetes had a fasting blood sugar level of below 125 mg/100 ml, and no person without diabetes had a level of above 115 mg/100 ml, there would be no problem of a tradeoff between sensitivity and specificity—a cutoff point of 120 would be perfect. This is a rare kind of situation; and where it does occur, the disease may be so obvious that no diagnostic testing is required.

Although tests of relatively high sensitivity and specificity do exist for some diseases, the scarcity of inexpensive, readily available tests that are both highly sensitive and highly specific means that it is often best to use a combination of tests when attempting to diagnose a particular disease. A highly sensitive test should be used first, almost guaranteeing the detection of all cases of the disease (albeit at the expense of including a number of false positive results), followed by a more specific test to eliminate the false positive results. In clinical situations there will also be practical and cost considerations that will play an important role in determining which tests are used at which stage of the diagnostic process.

PREDICTIVE VALUES

When the sensitivity of a test is known, it is possible to answer the question, "Given that a patient has the disease, what is the ability of the test to discover this?" When the specificity of a test is known, it is possible to answer the question, "Given that a patient is free of the disease, what is the ability of the test to discover this?" These are both the kinds of questions that an epidemiologist might ask when screening for a disease. The epidemiologist wants to know, for example, how good a test is at detecting the presence or absence of HIV infection, or what percentage of people with HIV infection will be detected with the test. But these are not the kinds of questions that the practicing physician or the patient wants answered; when faced with a test result, they want to know how likely it is that the disease really is present or absent. This is a different question altogether, and answering it requires knowledge of the **predictive values** of the test.

Positive predictive value

The **positive predictive value (PPV)** of a test is the proportion of positive results that are true positives, i.e., the likelihood that a person with a positive test result actually has the disease:

$$\text{PPV} = \frac{\text{number who test positive and have the disease } (TP)}{\text{total number who test positive } (TP + FP)}$$

Knowing a test's PPV allows one to answer the question "Given that the patient's test result is positive, how likely is it that he really has the disease?" This is the kind of information that a patient who tests positive (for HIV, for example) wants to know.

Negative predictive value

The **negative predictive value (NPV)** of a test is the proportion of negative results that are true negatives, i.e., the likelihood that a person with a negative result truly does not have the disease:

$$\text{NPV} = \frac{\text{number who test negative and do not have the disease } (TN)}{\text{total number who test negative } (FN + TN)}$$

Knowing a test's NPV allows one to answer the question "Given that the test result is negative, how likely is it that the disease really is absent?" Once again, this is the kind of information a patient is concerned about.

Whereas the sensitivity and specificity of a test depend only on the characteristics of the test itself and can be stated for any given test, *predictive values vary according to the prevalence (or underlying probability) of the disease.* Consequently, predictive values cannot be determined without prior knowledge of the prevalence of the disease. They are not qualities of the test *per se*, but are a function of the test's characteristics *and* of the setting in which it is being used.

The higher the prevalence of a disease in the population, the higher the PPV and the lower the NPV of a test for it. If a disease is rare, even a very specific test may have a low PPV because it produces a large number of false positive results. This is an important consideration because many new tests are first used in hospital populations, in which a given disease may be quite common. Therefore, a test may produce only a few false positive results at first. But when the test is used in the general population, in which the disease may be quite rare, it may produce an unacceptably high proportion of false positive results.

An example will make the relationship between predictive values and prevalence clearer:

In a community with a population of 10,000 people, of whom 10 are HIV-positive, the prevalence of HIV infection is 10 in 10,000, or 0.1%. If a test for HIV is 90% sensitive and 99% specific, the results of a community-wide screening program will be as shown in Table 7-2.

Table 7-2

HIV INFECTION

		Present	Absent
TEST RESULT	Positive	9 (TP)	100 (FP)
	Negative	1 (FN)	9890 (TN)

Because the test is 90% sensitive, 9 of the 10 people with HIV are detected; because it is 99% specific, 99% of the uninfected population, or 9890 people, are correctly identified as being free of the virus, leaving 100 false positive results.

The PPV of the test is $TP \div (TP + FP)$, or $9 \div (9 + 100)$, which is approximately equal to 0.08. This means that there is only an 8% chance that a person with a positive test result actually has the virus! On the other hand, the NPV is $TN \div (FN + TN)$, or $9890 \div (1 + 9890) = 0.9999$, meaning that a person with a negative test can be virtually 100% sure that he or she does not have the virus.

If there were an equally sensitive (90%) and specific (99%) test for hypertension, and 1000 people in this population were hypertensive, the prevalence would be 1000 per 10,000, or 10%. The results of a screening program for hypertension in the community would be as shown in Table 7-3.

Since the test is 90% sensitive, 900 of the 1000 hypertensive people are detected. Because the test is 99% specific, 99% of the 9000 normotensive people, or 8910 people, will be correctly classified, leaving 90 false positive results.

The PPV of this test is $TP \div (TP + FP)$, or $900 \div 990$, which is approximately equal to 0.91, meaning that there is a 91% chance that a person with a positive test result actually is hypertensive. The NPV of the test is $TN \div (FN + TN)$, or $8910 \div 9010$, or approximately 0.99, meaning that there is a 99% chance that a person with a negative test result is indeed normotensive.

Table 7-3

HYPERTENSION

		Present	Absent
T E S T **R E S U L T**	Positive	900 (*TP*)	90 (*FP*)
	Negative	100 (*FN*)	8910 (*TN*)

The enormous difference between the PPV of the test for hypertension (91%) and the PPV of the HIV test (8%) is entirely due to the different prevalences of the two diseases, as the two tests are identical in terms of their sensitivity and specificity. Notice that as the prevalence of the disease increases, PPV *increases* while NPV *decreases* (although only slightly in this example).

Because the PPV increases as the prevalence of the disease increases, one way of improving a test's PPV, and hence avoiding a large number of false positive results, is to restrict its use to high-risk members of the population. For example, if it were decided to use the HIV test only on the 10% of the population who are at the highest risk for HIV, the results might be as shown in Table 7-4.

Table 7-4

HIV INFECTION

		Present	Absent
T E S T **R E S U L T**	Positive	9 (*TP*)	10 (*FP*)
	Negative	1 (*FN*)	980 (*TN*)

Because all 10 HIV infections occur among members of this high-risk group, and because the test is 90% sensitive, 9 out of the 10 people with HIV are correctly identified, as before. Because the test is 99% specific, 99% of the 990 uninfected people, or 980 people, are correctly identified, leaving 10 false positive results.

The PPV of the test, $TP \div (TP + FP)$, is now $9 \div 19$, or 0.47 (47%), which is a vast improvement on the previous figure of 8%. The NPV of the test, $TN \div (TN + FN)$, is $980 \div 981$, or approximately 0.99, so it is essentially unchanged. Note how the PPV of the test has been enormously improved by limiting its use to high-risk members of the population.

Appendix 1: Statistical Symbols

Symbols are listed in order of their appearance in the text.

X A single element

N Number of elements in a population

n Number of elements in a sample

p The probability of an event occurring. In reports of statistical significance, p is the probability that the result could have been obtained by chance — i.e., the probability that a type I error is being made

q The probability of an event not occurring; equal to $(1 - p)$

f Frequency

C Centile (or percentile) rank; *or* confidence level

Mo Mode

Mdn Median

μ Population mean

$\overline{X}$ Sample mean

$\sum$ The sum of

x Deviation score

σ^2 Population variance

S^2 Sample variance

σ Population standard deviation *(SD)*

S Sample standard deviation *(SD)*

z The number of standard deviations by which a single element in a normally distributed population lies from the population mean; *or* the number of standard errors by which a random sample mean lies from the population mean

$\mu_{\overline{x}}$ The mean of the random sampling distribution of means

$\sigma_{\overline{x}}$ Standard error or standard error of the mean (standard deviation of the random sampling distribution of means) [*SEM* or *SE*]

$s_{\overline{x}}$ Estimated standard error (estimated standard error of the mean)

t The number of estimated standard errors by which a random sample mean lies from the population mean

df Degrees of freedom

α The criterion level at which the null hypothesis will be accepted or rejected; the probability of making a type I error

β Probability of making a type II error

F A ratio of variances

χ^2 Chi-square; a test of proportions

r Correlation coefficient

ρ Rho; Spearman rank order correlation coefficient

r^2 Coefficient of determination

b Regression coefficient; the slope of the regression line

Appendix 2 – Review Exercise Answers

CHAPTER 1

1. If $\overline{X} = 40$ and $X = 45$, x (the deviation score of the element X) is **+5**.

2. If $\overline{X} = 60$ and $X = 40$, x (the deviation score of the element X) is **–20**.

3. If $\mu = 37$ and $X = 29$, x (the deviation score of the element X) is **–8**.

4. The formula for variance in a sample is $S^2 = \dfrac{\sum(X-\overline{X})^2}{n}$ or $\dfrac{\sum x^2}{n}$

5. The formula for variance in a population is $\sigma^2 = \dfrac{\sum(X-\mu)^2}{N}$ or $\dfrac{\sum x^2}{n}$

6. The formula for standard deviation in a sample is the **square root** of the formula for sample variance in Answer 4; it is therefore symbolized by S.

7. The formula for standard deviation in a population is the **square root** of the formula for population variance in Answer 5; it is therefore symbolized by σ.

8. The proportion of any normal distribution that lies within approximately $\pm 1\sigma$ of μ is **.68**, or **68%**.

9. The proportion of any normal distribution that lies within approximately $\pm 2\sigma$ of μ is **.95**, or **95%**.

10. The proportion of any normal distribution that lies within approximately $\pm 3\sigma$ of μ is **.997**, or **99.7%**.

11. In a normal distribution, if $\mu = 10$, $\sigma = 2$, and $X = 12$, the z score of X is **+1**, because the score of 12 lies one standard deviation above the population mean.

12. In a normal distribution, if $\mu = 10$, $\sigma = 2$, and $X = 6$, the z score of X is **–2**, because the score of 6 lies two standard deviations below the population mean.

13. In a normal distribution, if $\mu = 10$ and $\sigma = 2$, the proportion of the distribution falling between 8 and 12 is **.68** or **68%**, because 8 and 12 are each one standard deviation away from the population mean.

14. In a normal distribution, if $\mu = 100$ and $\sigma = 20$, the proportion of the distribution falling between 60 and 140 is **.95**, or **95%**, because 60 and 140 are each two standard deviations away from the population mean.

15. In a normal distribution, if $\mu = 50$ and $\sigma = 10$, the probability of a randomly selected element having a score of above 70 is **.025**. This is because a score of 70 lies two standard deviations above the mean, and 95% of the distribution lies *within* two standard deviations of the mean; therefore, 5% of the distribution lies outside this 95% area — half of this 5% above a score of 70 and half of it below a score of 30. Therefore, 2.5% lies above a score of 70.

CHAPTER 2

1.   The standard deviation of the random sampling distribution of means is the **standard error**.

2.   The formula for the standard deviation of the random sampling distribution of means, better known as standard error, is $\sigma_{\overline{X}} = \dfrac{\sigma}{\sqrt{n}}$

3.   The z score of a random sample mean is expressed in terms of the number of **standard errors** by which it lies above or below the population mean.

4.   If $\overline{X} = 40$, $\mu = 50$, and $\sigma_{\overline{X}} = 5$, **z = -2**, because 40 lies 2 standard errors below μ.

5.   If $\overline{X} = 100$, $\mu = 85$, and $\sigma_{\overline{X}} = 7.5$, **z = +2**, because 100 lies 2 standard errors above μ.

6.   If $\sigma = 30$ and $n = 36$, $\sigma_{\overline{X}} = \mathbf{5}$, using the formula in Answer 2.

7.   If $\mu = 100$ and $\sigma_{\overline{X}} = 15$, the probability that a random sample drawn from this population will have a mean of between 70 and 130 is **.95**, because 130 and 70 are each 2 standard errors from μ.

8.   If $\sigma = 50$ and $n = 25$, $\sigma_{\overline{X}} = \mathbf{10}$, using the formula from Answer 2.

9.   If $\mu = 200$ and $\sigma = 50$, the probability that a random sample ($n = 25$) will have a mean above 210 or below 190 is **.32**. This is because 190 and 210 are each one standard error from the population mean (the standard error is 10, as determined in Answer 8); therefore, 68% (.68) of the distribution lies between 190 and 210, leaving 32% (.32) in the two tails of the curve above 210 and below 190.

10. If $\mu = 200$ and $\sigma = 50$, 95% of sample means ($n = 25$) would lie between **180 and 220**. This is because 95% of the random sampling distribution of means lies between ±2 standard errors of the population mean, and the standard error is 10 (as determined in Answer 8).

11. If μ is unknown, $\sigma = 50$, $\overline{X} = 200$, and $n = 25$, we can be 95% confident that μ lies between **180 and 220**. The formula (when z is used) for 95% confidence limits is $C = \overline{X} \pm z\sigma_{\overline{X}}$ — and the appropriate value for z is approximately 2, because 95% of the random sampling distribution of means lies between ±2 standard errors of the population mean. The standard error, $\sigma_{\overline{X}}$, is 10 (as determined in Answer 8).

12. If μ is unknown, $\sigma = 50$, $\overline{X} = 200$, and $n = 100$, we can be 95% confident that μ lies between **190 and 210**. This answer is obtained in the same way as the answer to Question 11, except that the standard error is now 5, not 10, due to the increase in sample size. *Note that the width of the confidence interval in Answer 11 has been halved by increasing the sample size fourfold, from 25 to 100.*

13. If μ is unknown, $\sigma = 50$, $\overline{X} = 200$, and $n = 400$, we can be 95% confident that μ lies between **195 and 205**. This answer is obtained in the same way as the answer to Question 12, except that the standard error is now 2.5, not 5, due to the additional increase in sample size. *Note that the width of the confidence interval in Answer 11 has been divided by four by increasing the sample size 16-fold, from 25 to 400.*

14. When $\sigma_{\overline{X}}$ (standard error) is not known, it is estimated by **estimated standard error, $s_{\overline{X}}$**.

15. The formula for standard error is $\sigma_{\overline{x}} = \dfrac{\sigma}{\sqrt{n}}$; the formula for estimated standard error is

$$s_{\overline{x}} = \frac{S}{\sqrt{n-1}}$$

16. When standard error is known, z scores are used to determine proportions of the normal distribution. When standard error is not known, z scores are replaced by **t scores**.

17. To calculate standard error, σ (population standard deviation) must be known. Instead of σ, only S (sample standard deviation) is required to calculate estimated standard error.

18. If $S = 12$ and $n = 10$, $s_{\overline{x}}$ is **4**, as calculated by the formula in Question 2.

19. If $S = 14$ and $n = 50$, $s_{\overline{x}}$ is **2**, as calculated by the formula in Question 2.

20. If $S = 3$ and $n = 82$, $s_{\overline{x}}$ is **⅓**, as calculated by the formula in Question 2.

21. If $\overline{X} = 46$, $\mu = 50$, and $s_{\overline{x}} = 2$, the t value corresponding to the sample mean is **–2**, because $\overline{X}$ is 2 estimated standard errors below the population mean.

22. If $\overline{X} = 12.4$, $\mu = 10.8$, and $s_{\overline{x}} = 0.8$, the t value corresponding to the sample mean is **+2**, because $\overline{X}$ is 2 estimated standard errors above the population mean.

23. If $n = 12$, $df = $ **11**, because df is $n - 1$ (for the purposes of answering questions at the level required by USMLE; in more advanced contexts df may take other values).

24. If $\overline{X} = 60$, $n = 26$, and $S = 10$, the 95% confidence limits for the estimate of μ are **55.88 and 64.12** (given that t_{25} for 95% of the distribution is 2.060). This answer is obtained by calculating $s_{\overline{x}}$ (estimated standard error) using the formula in Question 2, which gives the value of $s_{\overline{x}} = 2$, and then using the formula for confidence limits, $C = \overline{X} \pm ts_{\overline{x}}$. Note that the appropriate t value for 95% confidence limits will generally be in the region of 2; an approximate answer to this question would be 56 and 64, and could be given without knowing the exact value of t_{25}.

25. If $\overline{X} = 90$, $n = 63$, $s_{\overline{x}} = 4$, and t for a df of 62 and 95% of the distribution is 2.0, the 95% confidence limits for the estimate of the population mean are **82 and 98**. This answer is found in the same way as the answer to Question 24, except that $s_{\overline{x}}$ (estimated standard error) does not need to be calculated because it is already given.

CHAPTER 3

1. The null hypothesis H_0 is $\mu = 8$.

2. The alternative hypothesis H_A is $\mu \neq 8$. The alternative hypothesis is simply the logical alternative to the null hypothesis.

3. A directional alternative hypothesis could be used, and would therefore permit a one-tailed test, **only when results in a single direction are of interest, and when the possibility of the results being in the opposite direction is of no interest or consequence to the researcher.** In the present example, this means that a directional hypothesis could only be used if the student could legitimately claim that he is only interested in discovering if interns get less sleep than the general population, and that it would be of no interest or consequence at all if they

actually get *more* sleep than the general population — which is not a claim that could be made in this study.

4.   Sample mean $\overline{X} = \dfrac{\sum X}{n} = \dfrac{70}{10} = \mathbf{7}$

5.   Sample variance $S^2 = \dfrac{\sum x^2}{n} = \dfrac{83}{10} = \mathbf{8.3}$

6.   Estimated standard error $s_{\overline{x}} = \dfrac{S}{\sqrt{n-1}} = \dfrac{2.88}{\sqrt{9}} = \mathbf{0.96, \ or \ approximately \ 1}$

7.   Because estimated standard error is approximately 1, t_{calc} is **approximately –1**, because the sample mean (7) lies approximately 1 estimated standard error below the hypothesized population mean (8).

8.   If t_{crit} for $df = 9$ and $\alpha = .05$ is ±2.262, the null hypothesis must therefore be **accepted**, because t_{calc} does not exceed t_{crit}.

9.   The most straightforward way of improving the power of this test is to **increase the sample size**; this will reduce the estimated standard error, and thus increase t_{calc}, making it more likely that t_{calc} will fall beyond t_{crit}.

10.   **A *t*-test can still be used** even if interns' hours of sleep do not form a normal distribution, *provided that* the sample is a random one. The central limit theorem states that the means of random samples are elements in a normal distribution (which is the random sampling distribution of means), irrespective of the shape of the underlying population distribution.

11.   If this test was not powerful enough to detect a real difference between the interns' mean number of hours of sleep and that of null hypothesis, a **type II (false positive) error** is being made — the null hypothesis is being falsely accepted.

12.   The best estimate of the mean number of hours of sleep of the population of all interns is **7**.

13.   The approximate 95% confidence limits of this estimate are calculated according to the formula $C = \overline{X} \pm ts_{\overline{x}}$; they are therefore 7 ± (2.262 × 0.96) = **5 and 9** approximately (4.828 and 9.172 exactly).

References

Barnes DM: Promising results halt trial of anti-AIDS drug. *Science* 234: 15–16, 1986.

Herbst AL, Ulfelder H, Poskanzer DC: Adenocarcinoma of the vagina: Association of maternal stilbestrol therapy with tumor appearance in young women. *N Engl J Med* 284: 878–881, 1971.

Hill OW Jr: Rethinking the "significance" of the rejected null hypothesis. *Am Psychol* 45: 667–668, 1990.

Kupfersmid J: Improving what is published: A model in search of an editor. *Am Psychol* 43: 635–642, 1988.

Lipid Research Clinics Program: The Coronary Primary Prevention Trial: Design and implementation. *J Chronic Dis* 32: 609–631, 1979.

Rubin DH, Krasnilkoff PA, Leventhal JM, et al: Effect of passive smoking on birth-weight. *Lancet* ii: 415–417, 1986.

Zito RA, Reid PR: Lidocaine kinetics predicted by indocyanine green clearance. *N Engl J Med* 298: 1160–1163, 1978.